Student Study Guide

for use with

Abnormal Psychology
Clinical Perspectives on Psychological Disorders

Fifth Edition

Richard P. Halgin
University of Massachusetts-Amherst

Susan Krauss Whitbourne
University of Massachusetts-Amherst

Prepared by

Barbara Bowman
Washburn University
Topeka, Kansas

Boston   Burr Ridge, IL   Dubuque, IA   Madison, WI   New York   San Francisco   St. Louis
Bangkok   Bogotá   Caracas   Kuala Lumpur   Lisbon   London   Madrid   Mexico City
Milan   Montreal   New Delhi   Santiago   Seoul   Singapore   Sydney   Taipei   Toronto

The *McGraw·Hill* Companies

McGraw-Hill Higher Education

Student Study Guide for use with
Abnormal Psychology
Richard P. Halgin and Susan Krauss Whitbourne

1 2 3 4 5 6 7 8 9 0 QPD/QPD 0 9 8 7 6 5

ISBN-13: 978-0-07-320897-8
ISBN-10:   0-07-320097-3

www.mhhe.com

Table of Contents

Preface

This *Student Study Guide* continues the tradition set in the first four editions of **Abnormal Psychology** by Richard P. Halgin and Susan Krauss Whitbourne. This *Study Guide* helps you make efficient use of study time by organizing the material into segments that test your general knowledge of each chapter as well as assess specific concepts and issues.

Clear and Innovative Study Elements

The first page of each chapter, *Chapter at a Glance*, provides an overview of the chapter in a visual context. *Learning Objectives* guide you through the text, while *Review at a Glance* fill-in-the-blank sections test your specific knowledge of the main points in the chapter. Games, matching, and short-answer questions address the main chapter headings. These exercises reinforce the text's emphasis on blending history, theory, and application.

Focus on Critical Thinking and Evaluating Research

A strong element of this book is its focus on a case examined in detail in each chapter, *From the Case Files of Dr. Sarah Tobin.* Another feature is a section called *Focusing on Research* that asks you to evaluate the research methods and conclusions reported in text boxes.

Answers to Questions

The *Study Guide* provides answers to all objective questions in the guide as well as rejoinders for the comprehensive, multiple-choice reviews at the end of each chapter. In the rejoinders, you are given the right answer as well as the reason why the other answers are incorrect or incomplete. General answers are provided for the *From the Case Files of Dr. Sarah Tobin, Focusing on Research*, and other activities, but they are not intended to limit the direction that you may go in your thinking and evaluation.

Suggestions for Study

You have probably developed your own way of studying and using study aids like this *Study Guide*, but here are some suggestions for an effective way to learn from the material in this text.

1. Prior to reading the textbook chapter, review the learning objectives in the *Study Guide* and glance at the *Review at a Glance* feature.
2. Before you read each main section of the text, find the *Study Guide* components that relate to that section, and read them over before you read the text. Then complete each activity after you read each section in the text.
3. Before you read the text boxes, look over the *Focusing on Research* and *Social Context* activities in the Study Guide. After reading each of the boxes, complete these activities.

4. After you complete the chapter, complete *Review at a Glance*. Then turn to the *From the Case Files of Dr. Sarah Tobin* and see how the text material helps you better understand the case. Test your comprehensive knowledge by completing the multiple-choice questions at the end of each *Study Guide* chapter.
5. You can check all of your answers as you go along by referring to the answer key at the end of each chapter.
6. Always go back to the text, and reexamine material where your answers were inadequate. Do not settle for anything less than a thorough understanding of the text materials.

Multimedia Study Aides

Online Learning Center
The Student Online Learning Center houses an array of chapter-by-chapter study tools that complement this guide including detailed chapter outlines, learning objectives, key word flash cards, self-quizzes, and Internet exercises. Explore all these options and more at www.mhhe.com/halgin5.

Making the Grade Student CD-ROM
Packaged free with each copy of the text, this CD-ROM is designed to help students perform at their best. It contains practice quizzes for each text chapter, a learning style assessment, study skills primer, guide to electronic research, and a link to the text Web site.

While the general goal of this *Study Guide* is to help you master the material, it has been designed in a way that encourages you to be an active participant in your learning. Most students consider an Abnormal Psychology course to be one of the most interesting and rewarding of all undergraduate psychology courses. Your text is an excellent foundation for this experience. This *Study Guide* is a useful, challenging, and engaging companion that will enhance your understanding of psychological disorders.

Special thanks go to Elaine Cassel, who devised the many interesting word puzzles and similar learning features found in this guide. Thanks also to Mary Lee Harms, whose editorial encouragement and expertise made this an enjoyable project to work on.

Dr. Barbara Bowman
Washburn University
Topeka, Kansas

CHAPTER 1
UNDERSTANDING ABNORMALITY: A LOOK AT HISTORY AND RESEARCH METHODS

CHAPTER AT A GLANCE

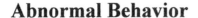

Abnormal Behavior

What Causes It?
Biological Causes
Psychological Causes
Sociocultural Causes

What Are Its Effects?
Impact on the Individual
Impact on the Family
Impact on the Community
Impact on Society

What Is It?
Distress
Impairment
Risk to Self and Others
Socially & Culturally Unacceptable
Behavior
Challenges Involved in
Characterizing Abnormal Behavior

Abnormal Psychology

**What Are Its Research
Methods?**
The Scientific Method
The Experimental Method

What Is Its History
Prehistoric Times
Ancient Greece and Rome
The Middle Ages and Renaissance
Europe and the United States in the 1700s
The 1800s to the 1900s
The Late Twentieth Century

Learning Objectives

1.0   What Is Abnormal Behavior?
     1.1   Recognize the difficulties of defining abnormal behavior because it overlaps with "normal" behavior.
     1.2   Contrast the view of abnormal behavior as deviation from the average with the view of abnormal behavior as deviation from the optimal.
     1.3   Define abnormal behavior as a concept that incorporates biological, psychological, and sociocultural dimensions.
     1.4   Discuss the challenges involved in characterizing abnormal behavior.
     1.5   Discuss the importance of the biopsychosocial perspective.
     1.6   Discuss the diathesis-stress model.

2.0   Abnormal Psychology throughout History
     2.1   Recognize the influence of beliefs about possession on prehistoric approaches to psychological disorders.
     2.2   Indicate how the beliefs of Hippocrates and Galen contributed to a scientific approach to understanding abnormal behavior.
     2.3   Explain the return in the Middle Ages to the belief that abnormal behavior is caused by demonic or spiritual possession, and how this belief was reflected in the treatment of the mentally ill.
     2.4   Describe the reform movement in Europe and the United States in the 1700s and the contributions of Chiarugi, Pinel, Tuke, Rush, and Dix.
     2.5   Explain the contributions of psychiatrists such as Greisinger and Kraepelin to contemporary medical approaches to treating the mentally ill.
     2.6   Describe the influence of Freud's psychoanalytic treatment of psychological disorders and the impact of its predecessors such as Braid, Mesmer, Liébault, Bernheim, and Charcot.
     2.7   Indicate how somatic treatments such as psychosurgery and electroconvulsive therapy were used and abused as treatment methods for those institutionalized.
     2.8   Explain the pros and cons of the deinstitutionalization movement and the components of successful community treatment programs.

3.0   Research Methods in Abnormal Psychology
     3.1   Describe the essential elements of the scientific method, including observation, hypothesis formation, and sampling.
     3.2   Explain the experimental method, and describe the concepts of independent and dependent variables, placebos, treatment and control groups, double-blind technique, the quasi-experimental design, and demand characteristics.
     3.3   Discuss the correlational method and define negative and positive correlations.
     3.4   Outline the survey method, and distinguish prevalence from incidence.
     3.5   Describe the case study method.
     3.6   Describe the pragmatic case study method.
     3.7   Indicate how the single-subject study is conducted, and how the multiple baseline technique is used in this type of research.
     3.8   Explain the logic and procedures involved in studies of genetic influence, including twin studies, adoption studies, cross-fostering studies, biological marker studies, and genetic mapping research.

4.0   The Human Experience of Psychological Disorders
     4.1   Explain the concepts of stigma and distress as they apply to an individual with a psychological disorder.
     4.2   Indicate how psychological disorders affect the individual, the family, community, and

society.
5.0   Chapter Boxes
     5.1   Discuss cultural variations in defining what is "abnormal" behavior.
     ~~5.2~~   Describe the importance of the study in which psychologists disguised themselves as psychiatric patients and sought admission to a hospital.
     ~~5.3~~   Discuss some of the key ideas in the case of Kelsey Grammar.

Identifying Historical Periods

Put the letter corresponding to the historical period in the blank next to each approach to psychological disorder:

P	=	Prehistoric	S	=	1700s
A	=	Ancient Greece and Rome	E	=	1800s to 1900s (approximately to 1950)
M	=	Middle Ages and Renaissance	T	=	Late Twentieth century (1950 and later)

Period	Approach to Psychological Disorders
1. _____	Reliance on superstition, alchemy, and astrology as explanations of psychological disorders.
2. _____	Emphasis on dysfunction of the brain as the cause of psychological disorder.
3. _____	First documented recognition of the role of emotional disturbances in causing psychological disorders.
4. _____	Use of mesmerism to redistribute disturbed bodily fluids thought to cause psychological disorder.
5. _____	First reform efforts made to remove patients from chains and other physical restraints.
6. _____	Punishment and execution of people thought to be witches.
7. _____	Development of managed care as an approach to outpatient treatment.
8. _____	Widespread use of electroconvulsive therapy and psychosurgery for treating psychological disorder.
9. _____	Large-scale release of patients from psychiatric hospitals into treatment sites in the community.
10. _____	Transformed poorhouses into asylums where psychologically disturbed individuals were punished.
11. _____	Rise of the medical model as an explanation of psychological disorder.
12. _____	Development of moral treatment as an approach to care for people with psychological disorder.
13. _____	Holes drilled in heads of people with psychological disorders as a method of releasing evil spirits.
14. _____	Growth of large publicly funded institutions designed for people with psychological disorders.

"Cattergories"

This puzzle is based on a popular board game in which contestants must think of an item in a specified category that begins with a certain letter. Each group below contains items with the same first letter. Provide the answer in the space provided.

P

_____ French hospital staff worker in the 1700s who influenced Pinel to free patients from their chains.

_____ Belief based in spirituality that the cause of psychological disorders lies in demonic control.

_____ Model of treatment for psychological disorders based on the notion of unconscious determinants.

_____ Control condition in an experiment in which subjects mistakenly believe they are receiving treatment.

_____ Entire group of people sharing a characteristic of interest to a researcher, from which a sample is derived.

S

_____ Negative label that is applied to people with who have been diagnosed with psychological disorders.

_____ Approach to investigation that involves observations, hypothesis testing, and controls.

_____ Englishman living in the 1500s who challenged the belief that demonic possession caused psychological disorder.

_____ Twentieth-century American psychiatrist who claims that mental illness is a "myth."

_____ Criterion of psychological disorders that focuses on violation of norms and potential harm to others.

H

_____ Greek philosopher who proposed that an imbalance of bodily fluids produced psychological disorder.

_____ Term coined by English physician Braid to describe the process of inducing a trance in an individual.

_____ Disorder treated by Freud and Breuer in which psychological problems are expressed in physical form.

_____ Prediction of a certain outcome in an experiment

Matching

Put the letter from the right-hand column corresponding to the correct match in the blank next to each item in the left-hand column.

1. ____ Research method in which the association is observed between two variables.
2. ____ Group in an experiment that does not receive the treatment being tested.
3. ____ Researcher who conducted a study in which "pseudopatients" were admitted to psychiatric hospitals.
4. ____ In an experiment, the variable whose value is observed after the manipulation is performed.
5. ____ Research method in which each person is studied in both the experimental and control conditions.
6. ____ Physician who, in the mid-1500s, criticized the prevailing view that psychological disorders were caused by demonic possession.
7. ____ American living in the 1800s who was an influential reformer of treatment of psychologically disturbed people.
8. ____ British psychiatrist who proposed that people who follow society's norms are more disturbed than those who refuse to do so.
9. ____ In an experiment, the variable whose value is set by the researcher.
10. ____ Treatment method discovered by Freud and Breuer in the case of Anna O. in which the client talks about emotional conflicts.
11. ____ Roman physician who studied psychological disorder through experimental, scientific methods.
12. ____ General name for the type of research method in which the investigator attempts to establish cause-effect relations.
13. ____ Group in an experiment that receives the treatment being tested.
14. ____ Type of study on genetic influences in which children of normal parents are adopted by parents with psychological disorders.
15. ____ Experimental approach in which neither the researcher nor the subject is aware of which condition the subject is in.

a. experimental method
b. Laing
c. double-blind
d. dependent variable
e. Weyer
f. cathartic
g. experimental group
h. Rosenhan
i. Dix
j. correlational
k. Galen
l. cross-fostering study
m. independent variable
n. single-subject design
o. control group

Short Answer

1. Place an "X" next to the word or name that does not belong:

    a. R. D. Laing
        Thomas Szasz
        William Greisinger
        David Rosenhan

    b. Dorothea Dix
        Vincenzo Chiarugi
        Philippe Pinel
        James Braid

    c. multiple baselines
        representativeness
        demand characteristics
        mesmerism

    d. pragmatic
        sanguine
        choleric
        phlegmatic

    e. Jean-Martin Charcot
        Benjamin Rush
        Josef Breuer
        Ambrose-Auguste Liébault

2. Match the period of history with the predominant orientation(s) to understanding and treating psychological disorders by filling in the blank with the letter representing the predominant orientation. Historical periods associated with more than one orientation have two blanks:

Period of History

____ Prehistoric times

____ Ancient Greece and Rome

____ Middle Ages and Renaissance

____ Europe and the U.S. in the 1700s
____ 1800s to 1900s

____ Late 20th century

Predominant orientation(s)

S = Scientific
H = Humanitarian
M = Mystical

3. Social Context: On Being Sane in Insane Places
   a. What led Rosenhan and his fellow pseudopatients to feel dehumanized?

   _____

   _____

   b. What did Rosenhan conclude when he was discharged as "in remission"?

   _____

   _____

   c. What are some of the criticisms of the Rosenhan study?

   _____

   _____

   d. How has the pendulum swung to an extreme that is opposite to the Rosenhan experience?

   _____

   _____

4. For each of the criteria for deviant behavior, describe the nature of the criterion, its applicability, and its limitations.

Criterion	Definition	Applicability	Limitations
Biological			
Psychological			
Sociocultural			

7

5. a. Describe four ways in which families are affected by the presence of a psychologically disturbed member:

_____
_____
_____
_____

    b. What has been an organized response of groups of families to these difficulties?

_____
_____
_____

    c. How are local communities affected by the presence of people with psychological disorder?

_____
_____
_____

6. a. What is the significance of the fact that monozygotic twins have a higher concordance rate of a disorder than dizpygotic twins?

_____
_____
_____

    b. Describe the major difference between an adoption study and a cross-fostering study:

_____
_____
_____

    c. What is the purpose for studies on biological markers?

_____
_____
_____

Focusing on Research

Answer the following questions concerning the Research Focus entitled "Are Creative People More Likely to Have Psychological Problems?"

1. What research method was used by Andreasen?

_____
_____
_____

2. Why was it necessary to include a group of people who were comparable in age, sex, and education to the writers?

_____

_____

_____

3. Why would it have been preferable for Andreasen to have conducted the study without knowing which subjects were creative writers and which were controls?

_____

_____

From the Case Files of Dr. Sarah Tobin: Thinking About Rebecca's Case

Answer the following questions about the case of Rebecca Hasbrouck.

1. Describe the symptoms of distress that Dr. Tobin observed in Rebecca.

_____

_____

2. How was Rebecca's life impaired as a result of her distress symptoms?

_____

_____

_____

3. In what way was Rebecca a threat to herself when she first met Dr. Tobin?

_____

_____

_____

4. What socially unacceptable behaviors had Rebecca engaged in since the onset of her illness?

_____

_____

_____

5. Explain how Rebecca's illness fits the diathesis-stress model of abnormal behavior.

_____

_____

_____

6. What was the course of Rebecca's hospital treatment, and what treatment and support did she receive on discharge?

_____

_____

_____

Review at a Glance

Test your knowledge by completing the blank spaces with terms from the chapter. If you need a hint, consult the chapter summary.

Abnormality can be defined according to four criteria: (1) _____, (2) _____, (3) _____, and (4) _____. In trying to understand the reasons people act and feel in ways that are regarded as abnormal, social scientists look at these dimensions: (5)_____, (6)_____, and (7)_____. The term (8) _____ characterizes the interaction among these three sets of influences. The (9) _____ model proposes that people are born with a predisposition that places them at risk for developing a psychological disorder.

Three recurring themes characterize the understanding and treatment of people with psychological disorders. They are the (10) _____, the (11) _____, and the (12) _____. The (13) _____ theme regards abnormality as due to demonic or spiritual possession. The (14) _____ theme regards abnormality as due to psychological or physical disturbances within the person. The (15) _____ regards abnormality as due to improper treatment by society.

Researchers use various methods to study the causes and treatment of psychological disorders. The (16) _____ method involves applying an objective set of methods for observing behavior, making a (17) _____ about the causes of behavior. In the (18) _____ method, the researcher alters the level of the (19) _____ and observes its effects on the (20) _____ variable. The (21) _____ method compares groups who differ on a predetermined characteristic. The (22) _____ method studies associations or relationships between variables. The (23) _____ method enables researchers to estimate the incidence and prevalence of psychological disorders. The (24) _____ method studies one individual intensively and conducts a careful and detailed analysis of the individual. In the (25) _____design, one person at a time is studied in experimental and control conditions.

True-False

Indicate whether the following statements are true or false.

1. If you want to prove what causes a psychological illness, conduct a correlational study.

    T　　　　　F

2. The dependent variable is adjusted or controlled by the experimenter.

    T   F

3. The control group consists of the subjects who receive a placebo.

    T   F

4. In the double-blind technique, only the person giving the treatment knows whether the subject is in the experimental group or the control group.

    T   F

5. Administering an electric shock to treat a mental disorder is known as trephining.

    T   F

6. The incidence of a disorder is a figure that tells us the number of people who have ever had a disorder at any given time or over a period of time.

    T   F

7. The prevalence of a disorder is the frequency of new cases within a given period of time.

    T   F

8. If you and your twin brother both suffer from depression, you may be, in research terms, discordant.

    T   F

9. The only thing that matters in a survey is the quality of answers you receive.

    T   F

10. The purpose of an adoption study is to see how well adopted children adjust to their adoptive

    T   F

Multiple Choice

1. When a person cannot function at an optimal or average level, they are considered to meet the criteria of
   a. distress.
   b. impairment.
   c. risk to self.
   d. socially unacceptable behavior.

2. Which American psychiatrist has argued that the concept of mental illness is a "myth" created in modern society and put into practice by the mental health profession?
   a. R. D. Laing
   b. David Rosenhan
   c. Thomas Szasz
   d. Marie Balter

3. Trephining is the term used for the procedure in which
   a. holes were drilled in a disturbed person's skull in order to release evil spirits.
   b. a ritual involving fire was used to invoke healthy mental energy as a replacement for unhealthy energy.
   c. blood was released from a person in the belief that an overabundance of blood caused unpredictable mood shifts.
   d. an individual was restrained in a "tranquilizer" chair.

4. Which theorist proposed that bodily fluids—black bile, yellow bile, phlegm, and blood—influence physical and mental health?
   a. Hippocrates
   b. Galen
   c. Eysenck
   d. Pinel

5. Which research method would most likely be used by a researcher interested in determining the relationship between IQ and level of anxiety?
   a. experimental
   b. case study
   c. single-subject design
   d. correlational

6. In 1792, an English Quaker named William Tuke established the York Retreat. Succeeding generations of Tuke's family carried on his work by using methods known as
   a. the "well-cure."
   b. the medical model.
   c. moral treatment.
   d. spiritual treatment.

7. The American Psychiatric Association was greatly influenced by Greisinger's 1845 book on the pathology and treatment of psychological disorders, which focused on the role in abnormal behavior of
   a. hormonal imbalances.
   b. demonic influence.
   c. early-life experience.
   d. brain dysfunction.

8. Anton Mesmer claimed that psychological cures could be brought about
   a. through the use of hypnosis.
   b. by redistributing the magnetic fluids in a person's body.
   c. through use of the cathartic method.
   d. by using psychoanalytic techniques.

9. The deinstitutionalization movement involved
   a. the restructuring of psychiatric institutions to make them more humane.
   b. the large-scale release of psychiatric clients into the community.
   c. the movement of psychiatric patients from public institutions to private institutions.
   d. the recognition that mental illness is a "myth."

10. A Chinese man who speaks to his dead relatives is an example of which aspect of abnormal behavior?
    a. attempt to fake schizophrenia
    b. genetic mapping
    c. the influence of religious beliefs
    d. mesmerism

11. A researcher tests the effectiveness of a medication so that neither the person administering nor the person receiving the treatment knows whether the subject is in the control or the experimental group. What is this technique?
    a. demand characteristic
    b. correlational
    c. experimental
    d. double-blind

12. Which of the following is considered to be a sociocultural criterion for defining abnormality?
    a. personal distress
    b. maladaptive behavior
    c. statistical deviation
    d. violated social conventions

13. A label that causes certain people to be regarded as different is referred to as a
    a. role.
    b. norm.
    c. stigma.
    d. diagnosis.

14. When did the scientific model of psychological disorders emerge?
    a. prehistoric times
    b. ancient Greece and Rome
    c. the Middle Ages
    d. the 20th century

15. Who is known as the founder of American psychiatry?
    a. Dorothea Dix
    b. Benjamin Rush
    c. William Tuke
    d. Clifford Beers

16. What was the most significant reason for the declining conditions in mental institutions during the later part of the reform period?
    a. overcrowding
    b. lack of funding
    c. undereducated staff
    d. re-emergence of spiritual explanations

17. Who was primarily responsible for reform in American mental institutions?
    a. Benjamin Rush
    b. Clifford Beers
    c. Dorothea Dix
    d. William Godding

18. Which of the following methods is most effective for determining cause and effect relationships?
    a. case study
    b. correlational
    c. survey method
    d. experimental

19. Which perspective on abnormality is based on the interaction of several sets of influences?
    a. humanitarian
    b. medical
    c. biopsychosocial
    d. supernatural

20. Which type of explanation of psychological disorders regards abnormal behavior as the product of possession by evil or demonic spirits?
    a. mystical
    b. scientific
    c. humanitarian
    d. psychological

21. The philosophy of Chiarugi, Pinel, and Tuke that people can, with the proper care, develop self-control over their own disturbing behaviors is referred to as
    a. psychotherapy.
    b. hypnosis.
    c. moral treatment.
    d. deinstitutionalization

22. The method of using suggestion to induce a trance state is called
    a. somnambulism.
    b. trephining.
    c. hypnotism.
    d. psychotherapy

23. The theory and system of practice that relies on the concepts of the unconscious mind, inhibited sexual impulses, early development, and the use of free association and dream analysis is called
    a. psychoanalysis
    b. hypnotherapy
    c. lobotomy
    d. person-centered theory

24. The variable whose level is adjusted or controlled by the experimenter is referred to as the variable.
    a. placebo
    b. dependent
    c. independent
    d. correlational

25. The attempt by biological researchers to identify the characteristics controlled by each gene is referred to as
    a. biological marking.
    b. cognitive mapping.
    c. genetic mapping.
    d. sensory gating.

Answers

IDENTIFYING HISTORICAL PERIODS

1. M	6. M	11. E
2. E	7. T	12. S
3. A	8. T	13. P
4. E	9. T	14. E
5. S	10. M	

"CATTERGORIES"

P	S	H
Pussin	Stigma	Hippocrates
Possession	Scientific	Hypnosis
Psychoanalysis	Scot	Hysteria
Placebo	Szasz	Hypothesis
Population	Sociocultural	Heraclitus

MATCHING

1. j	6. e	11. k

2.	o	7.	i	12.	a
3	h	8.	b	13.	g
4.	d	9.	m	14.	l
5	n	10.	f	15.	c

SHORT ANSWER

1. a. William Greisinger: Contemporary critics of medical model   2. M
    b. James Braid: 18th century reformers of treatment   S
    c. mesmerism: terms related to research methods   M & H
    d. pragmatic: The dispositions proposed by Hippocrates   H
    e. Benjamin Rush: Physicians who developed hypnosis   S
                                                                                      S & H

3. a. Staff did not seem to care about the patients' needs or personal issues. The staff did not believe what the patients said, although some of the other patients were suspicious of the true purpose of the study!
    b. There was a bias to err on the side of caution, and thus suspect illness even among healthy people.
    c. An ethical criticism was that Rosenhan used deception. He and his friends lied to the hospital staff about their symptoms. A methodological criticism was that there was no experimental control group. A diagnostic criticism was that staff had to believe the patients were seriously ill, since those patients reported very serious symptoms (hallucinations).
    d. While Rosenhan and friends had no trouble getting admitted, in more recent decades it is sometimes very difficult for patients who truly need help to be admitted.

4.

Criterion	Definition	Applicability	Limitations
Biological	Disorder or dysfunction in a part of the body or aspect of biological functioning.	Biological factors play important role in cause, expression, and treatment of abnormal behavior.	Not relevant to all disorders.
Psychological	Disorder of emotional state, intellect, memory, language use, adaptation, ability to satisfy personal needs; feelings of personal distress.	Feelings of unhappiness and maladjustment are useful indicators of dysfunction.	People may show maladaptive behavior but not necessarily feel distressed.
Sociocultural	Violation of social norms.	Situations in which people behave unacceptably or cause harm to others	Not every member of a society agrees in regards to what is "acceptable."

5. a. Feeling the pain of the affected member.
        Worrying that the affected member will be harmed.
        Experiencing the stigma of the affected family member.
        Feeling blamed by the mental health profession for the person's problems.
    b. Families have formed support and education groups such as the National Alliance for the Mentally Ill.
        Books have also been written that specifically concern family issues.
    c. Halfway houses and day treatment centers may need to be established for deinstitutionalized individuals. In the absence of sufficient treatment programs, psychologically disturbed people may become part of the homeless population of a community.

6. a. The disorder probably has a genetic basis because monozygotic twins have identical genetic inheritance.
    b. In an adoption study, a child of biologically disordered parents is adopted by parents who have no psychological disorder; in a cross-fostering study, a child of normal parents is adopted by parents who have psychological disorders.

c. In studies of biological markers, researchers attempt to understand the specific mechanisms involved in models of genetic transmission.

FOCUSING ON RESEARCH

1. Correlational, because she was investigating the relationship between two naturally occurring phenomena
2. A control group of people with comparable age, sex, and education was needed to rule out the possibility that any observed relationship between creativity and psychological disorder was due to factors other than the backgrounds of the writers. This was an important aspect of the study, because a higher rate of psychological disorder was observed in the "controls" than would be expected on statistical grounds.
3. Because Andreasen knew the identity of her subjects, it might have been difficult for her to evaluate her hypothesis objectively. However, the fact that Andreasen found a relationship between creativity and mood disorder (not schizophrenia, as she had predicted), suggests that her awareness of the subjects' identity did not bias her evaluation of their psychological status

FROM THE CASE FILES OF DR. SARAH TOBIN: THINKING ABOUT REBECCA'S CASE

Here are some suggestions for possible answers, not a comprehensive discussion of the topics.

1. Rebecca was disheveled, with dirty hair and torn and stained clothing. She was homeless, and said she wanted to return to the world she had left three years earlier.
2. Rebecca lost her career and her home after the illness that took her to such depths of despair. She heard voices that were not there and had delusions concerning the whereabouts of her husband and children.
3. Rebecca was a threat to herself because she was homeless and, at times, incoherent. She reported hearing voices.
4. Her joblessness, homelessness, unkempt and dirty physical appearance, hearing voices and having delusions.
5. Since her mother suffered from depression, Rebecca may have inherited a predisposition to depression (diathesis). The loss of her husband and children in an accident in which she survived led to her breakdown. She may have felt guilt for surviving (stress). Her mother and mother-in-law wanted nothing to do with her after the tragedy, so Rebecca was left without loved ones to grieve with (stress). The tragedy overwhelmed Rebecca, and she lost the ability to continue in her work.
6. During her hospital stay, Rebecca received a comprehensive physical and mental evaluation. She attended group therapy and had individual therapy. Dr. Tobin consulted with a social worker, who began to help Rebecca reconnect with her family and find her a place to live and employment. After two weeks in the hospital, Rebecca went to a halfway house for women who had suffered similar breaks with reality. After being there a month, she found an apartment and a new line of work that was less stressful. She continued in individual therapy with Dr. Tobin for a year.

REVIEW AT A GLANCE

1. distress
2. impairment
3. risk to self or others
4. behavior that deviates from social and cultural norms
5. biological
6. psychological
7. sociocultural
8. biopsychosocial
9. diathesis-stress model
10. mystical
11. scientific
12. humanitarian
13. mystical
14. scientific
15. humanitarian
16. scientific method
17. hypothesis
18. experimental
19. independent variable
20. dependent variable
21. quasi-experimental
22. correlational
23. survey
24. case study
25. single-subject design

TRUE-FALSE

1. False—Only an experiment can prove causation. Correlational studies may indicate a relationship between

variables, but not causation.

2. False—The independent variable is adjusted or controlled by the experimenter to study its effect on the dependent variable.

3. True—The experimental group receives the treatment.

4. False—Neither the person giving the treatment nor the subjects know who is getting the treatment.

5. False—Trephining was an ancient technique that involved drilling holes in the heads of people manifesting abnormal behavior.

6. False—Incidence is the frequency of new cases within a given period of time. See answer 7.

7. False—Prevalence of a disorder is a figure that indicates the number of people who have ever had a disorder at any given time or over a period of time. See answer 6.

8. False—You would be considered "concordant" for expressing the disorder, meaning that you both express it. If you were discordant, one of you would not have the disorder.

9. False—Among other things, number of people that respond to a survey, as well as the types of questions and how they are framed, are important indicators of a survey's research value.

10. False—Adoption studies attempt to determine what aspects of a person's makeup are genetic (from their biological parents) and what are environmental.

MULTIPLE CHOICE

1. The answer is (b). Distress (a) is more personal within the individual. Being unable to function well does not necessarily mean anyone is at risk (c); nor that what they are doing is socially unacceptable (d).

2. The answer is (c), Thomas Szasz. (a) R. D. Laing contended that modern society dehumanized the individual; (b) David Rosenhan conducted the research into mental institutions (that is discussed in your text); and (d)

3. The answer is (a). The other choices are also "treatments" used in the past, but (a) is the only one defined by the term *trephining*.

4. The answer is (a). (b) Galen conducted experiments on animals to understand human anatomy; (c) Eysenck is a contemporary theorist whose personality theory builds on Hippocrates' idea of bodily fluids; (d) Pinel was an eighteenth-century French reformer.

5. The answer is (d). The correlational method examines relationships between two variables. (a) The experimental method seeks to prove causation by using experimental and control groups; (b) case study is an in-depth study of one person; (c) single-subject design studies one person in both experimental and control conditions.

6. The answer is (c). (a) The "well-cure" is not a method of treatment; (b) the medical model treats mental illness with drugs or other medical means; (d) spiritual treatment relies on prayer and religious practices.

7. The answer is (d). Greisinger's book did not deal with (a), (b), or (c).

8. The answer is (b). (a) Hypnosis was espoused by Charcot; (c) Rush believed in the cathartic method; (d) Freud pioneered psychoanalytic techniques.

9. The answer is (b). The other answers are wrong because of the definition of the word *deinstitutionalization*. It means releasing people from institutions, not (a) making institutions more human; (c) privatizing institutions; or (d) making a statement about mental illness.

10. The answer is (c). (a) is wrong because suggesting that people who believe they commune with the dead are mentally ill is a sociocultural bias; (b) *genetic mapping* means identifying the human genes; (d) mesmerism was the technique of attempting to "redistribute" the body's "magnetic fluids" in an effort to treat mental illness.

11. The answer is (d). (a) Demand characteristic involves subjects trying to behave in the way they think will support the research hypothesis; (b) correlational studies examine relationships between variables and does not involved giving a treatment; (c) the experimental method relies on the double-blind technique to ensure maximum validity of research results.

12. The answer is (d). (a) and (b) are individual criteria; (c) is a scientific criterion.

13. The answer is (c). (a) involves behaving according to expectations; (b) is a behavioral standard; and (d) is the name given a disorder.

14. The answer is (b), as supported by historical texts.

15. The answer is (b). (a) Dorothea Dix sought to reform mental institutions to make them more humane; (c) William Tuke first proposed moral treatment; (d) Clifford Beers followed in Dix's path to continue reform of

psychiatric institutions.

16. The answer is (a). (b) and (c) Both lack of funding and undereducated staff contributed to declining conditions but were not as significant as overcrowding; (d) there was not a re-emergence of spiritual explanations for mental illness at the end of the reform period.

17. The answer is (c). (a) Benjamin Rush is considered the founder of American psychiatry; (b) Clifford Beers was involved in reform efforts as a result of Dix's pioneering efforts; and (d) William Godding felt there was an increasing prevalence of severe psychiatric disorders.

18. The answer is (d). Neither (a), (b), nor (c) can ever result in a determination of cause and effect between variables.

19. 19. The answer is (c). (a),and (d) are not perspectives on abnormality: (b) does not involve interaction with any other influence.

20. The answer is (c). (a) and (d) are not perspectives on abnormality; (b) does not involve interaction with any other influence.

21. The answer is (a). (b) explains disorders by empirical data; (c) is not an explanation of disorders; and(d) explains disorders as a function of individual cognitive and emotional processes.

22. The answer is (c). (a) involves methods to make the unconscious impulses surface; (b) involves being put into a trance; and (d) deinstitutionalization refers to the large-scale release of psychiatric patients from institutions into the community

23. The answer is (c). (a) is sleepwalking; (b) involved drilling holes in the head; and (d) does not include putting clients into a trance.

24. The answer is (a). (b) involves being put into a trance-like state; (c) is a surgical procedure; and (d) emphasizes client-therapist relationship.

25. The answer is (c). (b) is a measurement of the effect due to the independent variable; (a) is what the control group receives instead of the treatment; and (d) is a research method.

26. The answer is (c). (a) can lead to genetic mapping; (b) and (d) are not research methods or procedures.

CHAPTER 2
CLASSIFICATION AND TREATMENT PLANS

CHAPTER AT A GLANCE

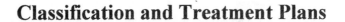

Classification and Treatment Plans

Diagnosis
Client's Symptoms
Diagnostic Criteria/Differential
Diagnosis
Final Diagnosis
Case Formulation
Cultural Formulation

DSM-IV-TR
Its Development
Definitions of "Mental Disorder"
Its Assumptions
The Five Axes

Treatment
Goals
Site
Modality
Theoretical Perspectives
Implementation
Treatment Course
Treatment Outcome

Learning Objectives

1.0   Psychological Disorder: Experiences of Client and Clinician
       1.1   Distinguish the concept of a client from that of a patient as the individual who is the focus of psychological treatment.
       1.2   Describe the prevalence of psychological disorders in the United States.
       1.3   Describe the types of clinicians who provide psychological treatment.

2.0   *The Diagnostic and Statistical Manual of Mental Disorders*
       2.1   Outline the history of the development of *DSM-IV-TR*.
       2.2   Define the term "mental disorder" as it is used in *DSM-IV-TR*.
       2.3   Explain the assumptions underlying the *DSM-IV-TR*, including the medical model, a theoretical orientation, categorical approach, and multiaxial system.
       2.4   Discuss the controversial issues and criticisms pertaining to the DSM.
       2.5   Define the five axes of *DSM-IV-TR*.
            Axis I: Clinical Disorders
            Axis II: Personality Disorders and Mental Retardation
            Axis III: General Medical Conditions
            Axis IV: Psychosocial and Environmental Problems
            Axis V: Global Assessment of Functioning

3.0   The Diagnostic Process
       3.1   Explain how the clinician obtains the client's reported symptoms.
       3.2   Indicate how the diagnostic criteria of *DSM-IV-TR* are used in identifying a possible diagnosis, including the role of the decision tree.
       3.3   Discuss the ways in which the clinician rules out differential diagnoses.
       3.4   Explain how the clinician arrives at a final diagnosis.
       3.5   Indicate how a case formulation is constructed.

4.0   Treatment Planning
       4.1   Contrast short- and long-term goals of treatment.
       4.2   Distinguish the treatment sites of psychiatric hospitals, outpatient clinics, halfway houses, and day treatment programs.
       4.3   Explain the various modalities of treatment, including individual psychotherapy, family therapy, group therapy, and milieu therapy.
       4.4   Discuss the role of the clinician's theoretical perspective as it influences the nature of treatment.
       4.5   Discuss how to determine the Best Approach to Treatment.

5.0   Treatment Implementation
       5.1   Indicate the roles of the clinician and client as they influence the course of treatment.
       5.2   Discuss the frustrations and possible limitations involved in providing effective psychological treatment.

6.0   Chapter Boxes
       6.1   Discuss the notion that the *DSM-IV-TR* unfairly labels people.
       ~~6.2~~   Highlight the significant factors from the life of actress Patty Duke.
       ~~6.3~~   Discuss how experts determine which treatments are effective.

Matching

Put the letter from the right-hand column corresponding to the correct match in the blank next to each item in the left-hand column.

1. ____ Consistency of measures or diagnoses.

2. ____ Term meaning the form in which psychotherapy is offered.

3. ____ Diagnostic dimension that applies to clinical syndromes.

4. ____ Illness seen in Latinos in which a frightening event causes the "soul" to leave the body, resulting in depression and somatic symptoms.

5. ____ Structured community-based treatment program similar to that found in a psychiatric hospital.

6. ____ *DSM* scale that rates an individual's overall health.

7. ____ Common term that refers to behavior involving loss of contact with reality.

8. ____ Accuracy of a diagnosis or measure.

9. ____ Approach to treatment in a psychiatric hospital in which the total environment is structured to be therapeutic.

10. ____ A client's likelihood of recovering from a disorder.

11. ____ Process through which a clinician systematically rules out alternative diagnoses.

12. ____ Axis in *DSM* for designating long-standing, maladaptive features of personality.

13. ____ Explanation of a client's psychological status that accompanies a diagnosis.

14. ____ Primary disorder for which the client is seeking treatment.

15. ____ Disorder found in Malaysia in which a man experiences a violent outburst, usually following an insult.

a. validity
b. modality
c. milieu therapy
d. differential diagnosis
e. Axis II of the *DSM*
f. susto
g. amok
h. case formulation
i. reliability
j. Axis I of the *DSM*
k. day treatment
l. principal diagnosis
m. psychosis
n. Global Assessment of Functioning
o. prognosis

Identifying the Axis

Put the Roman numeral corresponding to the axis on the DSM represented by each of the symptoms or characteristics below:

I   =   Clinical syndromes
II =   Personality disorders and mental retardation
III =   Physical disorders or conditions

IV =   Psychosocial and environmental problems
V   =   Global Assessment of Functioning

Axis	Symptoms or characteristics	Axis	Symptoms or characteristics
1. ____	Brain damage that interferes with memory	7. ____	Recent unemployment
2. ____	Extreme sadness, guilt, and suicidality	8. ____	Gastric ulcer
3. ____	Mental retardation	9. ____	Symptom severity ratings
4. ____	Death of a spouse	10. ____	Severe anxiety in social situations.
5. ____	Chronic bronchitis	11. ____	Deficient ability to carry out tasks of everyday living
6. ____	Personality characterized by constant dependency on others		

Short Answer

1. Explain the three main assumptions of the *DSM* regarding mental disorders:

Assumption about "mental disorder"	Explanation
The disorder is clinically significant.	
The disorder is reflected in a syndrome.	
The disorder is associated with present distress, impairment, or risk.	
The disorder is not a culturally sanctioned response.	

2. For each step of the diagnostic process, describe elements that the clinician must consider:

Step in diagnostic process	Elements that clinician considers
Client's reported symptoms	
Diagnostic criteria	
Differential diagnosis	
Final diagnosis	
Case formulation	

3. For each of the following treatment sites, describe the type of services provided and the reasons for referring clients to each site:

Treatment site	Type of service provided	Reasons for referral
Psychiatric hospital		
Outpatient treatment		
Halfway house		
Day treatment		

4. Answer the following questions about the process of implementing treatment for psychological disorders:

   a. What would lead a clinician to recommend family therapy rather than individual therapy?

   _____

   _____

   b. How does family therapy differ from group therapy?

   _____

   _____

   c. What is the role of a clinician's theoretical orientation in providing treatment?

   _____

   _____

d. How might the clinician's reactions to a client influence the course of treatment?

_____

_____

e. What is the client's role in the treatment process?

_____

_____

f. What are some of the obstacles that can interfere with successful outcomes of treatment?

_____

_____

5. Describe the aims of each successive edition of the *DSM*:

DSM Edition	Goal	Limitations
I		
II		
III		
III-R		
IV		

Focusing on Research

Answer the following questions concerning the Research Focus entitled "How Do Experts Determine Which Treatments Really Work?"

1. Compare and contrast the goals and research methods of *efficacy research* and *effectiveness research* in terms of analyzing psychotherapy.

_____

_____

_____

2. Briefly summarize Seligman's argument that *efficacy studies* don't tell the whole story about the value of psychotherapy.

_____

_____

_____

3. As a potential consumer of psychotherapy, which types of study would you pay most attention to and why?

_____

_____

_____

4. What are ESTs? According to Chamblis and Ollendick, what are some of the dangers in ignoring EST research?

_____

_____

_____

From the Case Files of Dr. Sarah Tobin: Thinking About Peter's Case

Answer the following questions about the case of Peter Dickinson.

1. Briefly list Peter's symptoms reported by Peter, his mother, and his brother, Don.

_____

_____

2. What symptoms did Dr. Tobin observe in Peter?

_____

_____

3. What was Dr. Tobin's diagnosis of Peter?

_____

_____

4. Describe the course of Peter's treatment, both in the hospital and after discharge.

_____

_____

5. Concerning the outcome of Peter's treatment, would you characterize his treatment as effective? Why or why not?

_____

_____

Review at a Glance

Test your knowledge by completing the blank spaces with terms from the chapter. If you need a hint, consult the chapter summary.

Nearly (1) _____ the population is afflicted with a diagnosable psychological disorder at some time in life. Approximately (2) _____ percent of these people seek professional help from clinicians, (3) _____ percent from other processional sources. The remainder turns to informal sources of support or goes without help. Clinicians are found within several professions, such as (4) _____, (5) _____, (6) _____, (7) _____, and (8) _____ counseling.

Clinicians and researchers use the (9) _____, which contains descriptions of all psychological disorders. In recent editions the authors have tried to meet the criterion of (10) _____ so that a given diagnosis will be consistently applied to anyone showing a particular set of symptoms. Researchers have also worked to ensure the (11) _____ of the classification system that that the various diagnoses represent real and distinct clinical phenomenon. The *DSM-IV-TR* is based on a (12) _____ model orientation in which disorders are viewed as (13) _____. Diagnoses are categorized in terms of relevant areas of functioning called (14) _____. Axis I includes (15) _____; Axis II, (16) _____; Axis III, (17) _____; Axis IV, (18) _____; and Axis V contains the (19) _____ scale.

The diagnostic process involves using all relevant information to arrive at a label that characterizes a client's disorder. After attending to a client's reported and observable symptoms, the clinician uses the *DSM-IV-TR* criteria and a strategy known as a (20) _____. The clinician rules out (21) _____ and tries to assign a (22) _____. After the diagnostic process, clinicians develop a (23) _____, in an effort to understand the processes and factors that might have influenced the client's current psychological status.

Once a diagnosis is determined, a (24) _____ plan is developed, which includes issues pertaining to (25) _____, (26) _____, and (27) _____. A (28) _____ is recommended. Possibilities include a (29) _____, (30) _____, (31) _____, (32) _____, or another appropriate setting. The treatment (33) _____ is specified, and may involve (34) _____, (35) _____, (36) _____, or (37) _____ therapy. After a plan is developed, clinicians implement treatment with particular attention to the fact that the (38) _____ is a crucial determinant of whether therapy will succeed.

Multiple Choice

1. A doctoral-level clinician who has been trained as a medical doctor is called a
   a. clinical psychologist.
   b. clinician.
   c. psychiatrist.
   d. neurophysiologist.

2. The *DSM* was developed to ensure that a given diagnosis would be consistently applied. This criterion is referred to as
   a. reliability.
   b. validity.
   c. predictability.
   d. base rate.

3. What is the commonly used term for behavior involving a person's loss of contact with reality?
   a. neurosis
   b. psychosis
   c. derealization
   d. syndrome

4. Upon admission to a psychiatric hospital for bizarre behavior, Carlos states that he has diabetes. This medical information would be noted on ___ of *DSM-IV-TR*.
   a. Axis I
   b. Axis II
   c. Axis III
   d. Axis IV

5. Matthew has recently been discharged from a psychiatric hospital and is moving to a facility with other discharged residents until ready to live independently. Such a facility is called a
   a. day treatment center.
   b. community mental health center.
   c. milieu therapy center.
   d. halfway house

6. In epidemiological research on racial differences in rates of psychological disorders, reports of higher rates among African Americans appear due to
   a. methodological problems.
   b. true racial differences.
   c. lack of recent data.
   d. prejudice by the researchers.

7. What is the term that refers to a client's likelihood of recovering from a disorder?
   a. prediction
   b. syndrome
   c. prognosis
   d. base rate

8. A collection of symptoms that together form a definable pattern is a
   a. diagnosis.
   b. syndrome.
   c. prognosis.
   d. disorder.

9. Which model does the *DSM* adhere to?
   a. psychoanalytic
   b. behavioral
   c. mystical
   d. medical

10. Axis II of the *DSM* is used for
    a. clinical syndromes.
    b. personality disorders and mental retardation.
    c. organic brain disorders.
    d. substance abuse disorders.

11. The process of ruling out possible alternative diagnoses is called
    a. differential diagnosis.
    b. compound diagnosis.
    c. assessment of functioning.
    d. multiaxial diagnosis.

12. An analysis of the client's development and the factors that may have influenced the client's current emotional state is called a
    a. diagnosis.
    b. prognosis.
    c. classification.
    d. case formulation.

13. What treatment site is usually recommended by a clinician when the client presents a risk of harming themselves or others?
    a. community mental health center
    b. psychiatric hospital
    c. halfway house
    d. outpatient treatment center

14. A man arrives one hour late for work every day because he is compelled to read every street sign on the road to his workplace. Which of the following components of a mental disorder is exemplified by his behavior?
    a. It reflects a behavioral syndrome.
    b. It is associated with impairment in life.
    c. It is a culturally sanctioned response.
    d. It reflects a serious risk.

15. The first step for a clinician in the diagnostic process involves
    a. ruling out differential diagnoses.
    b. planning a treatment strategy.
    c. reviewing the *DSM* criteria for disorders matching the client's symptoms.
    d. commencing the treatment program.

16. Roger is in the stage of therapy where he and his therapist are working on altering his long-standing patterns of dependent behavior. What phase of therapy is Roger in?
    a. immediate management
    b. assessment of objectives
    c. management of short-term goals
    d. management of long-term goals

17. An outpatient clinic that provides psychological services on a sliding fee scale and serves individuals who live in a certain geographic region is called a(n)
    a. halfway house.
    b. psychiatric hospital.
    c. community mental health center.
    d. asylum.

18. Structured programs in a community treatment facility that provides activities similar to those provided in a psychiatric hospital are called
    a. day treatment programs.
    b. CMHCs.
    c. asylums.
    d. halfway houses.

19. A treatment approach used in an inpatient psychiatric facility in which all facets of the environment are components of the treatment is referred to as _____ therapy.
    a. psychoanalytic
    b. person-centered
    c. milieu
    d. group

20. What is the current trend with regard to theoretical perspectives and treatment of psychological disorders?
    a. person-centered theory
    b. psychodynamic theory
    c. object relations theory
    d. the combination of elements from various orientations

Answers

MATCHING

1.	i		9.	c
2.	b		10.	o
3.	j		11.	d
4.	f		12.	e
5.	k		13.	h
6.	n		14.	l
7.	m		15.	g
8.	a			

IDENTIFYING THE AXIS

1.	I		
2.	I	7.	IV
3.	II	8.	III
4.	IV	9.	V
5.	III	10.	I
6.	II	11.	II

SHORT ANSWER

1.

Assumption about "mental disorder"	Explanation
The disorder is clinically significant.	Symptoms must be present to a significant degree and for a significant period of time.
The disorder is reflected in a syndrome.	Individual symptoms or problematic behaviors are not sufficient for diagnosis as a mental disorder.
The disorder is associated with present distress, impairment, or risk.	The behaviors or symptoms must involve personal or social cost.
The disorder is not a culturally sanctioned response.	The disorder is not expectable for one's society or culture.

2.

Step in diagnostic process	Elements that clinician considers
Client's reported symptoms	Compare the client's statement of problems with diagnostic terms and concepts.
Diagnostic criteria	Clarify the nature of the client's symptoms and attempt to match them with diagnostic criteria by following the decision tree.
Differential diagnosis	Rule out alternative diagnoses.
Final diagnosis	Provide diagnoses and ratings on the five axes of the *DSM*.
Case formulation	Place into perspective the client's diagnosis in the context of the client's life history.

3.

Treatment site	Type of service provided	Reasons for referral
Psychiatric hospital	24-hour inpatient treatment, which may include medical and psychotherapeutic interventions best offered in a setting with close monitoring and supervision.	Client at risk of harming self or others.
Outpatient treatment	Psychotherapy and counseling.	Hospitalization is a radical and expensive form of treatment and is not always needed.
Halfway house	Interaction with other deinstitutionalized clients and supervision by professional staff who can help clients develop skills needed for independent living.	Client is recently deinstitutionalized and is not yet ready for independent living.
Day treatment	Clients participate in structured activity similar to that offered in a hospital setting.	Client does not need to be hospitalized but needs structured support during the day.

4. a. The clinician determines that, although one person is the "patient," this person's difficulties reflect problems in the family as a whole.

b. In group therapy, participants are unrelated clients who work together to share their difficulties and problems in a setting where they can receive feedback, develop trust, and improve their interpersonal skills. In family therapy, the therapist works with related individuals as a system to help alleviate the distress of one member.

c. Clinicians are often trained with particular theoretical orientations that form the basis for the services they provide. However, most clinicians adapt their own perspective and combine it with elements of other perspectives to tailor their treatment to the needs of the individual client.

d. Each client stimulates a different reaction in the clinician, who must be alert to these reactions.

e. The client has the responsibility for presenting and clarifying the nature of his or her symptoms and reactions to therapy as it progresses and to implement changes suggested in treatment. These areas of responsibility can be complicated by the nature of therapy, which is highly personal and demanding, and by the nature of the client's psychological difficulties, which can interfere with the progress of therapy.

f. Client's unwillingness to change, financial constraints, refusal by another party to cooperate with therapy, and a variety of practical difficulties in the client's life.

5.

DSM Edition	Goal	Limitations
I	Search for a standard set of diagnostic criteria.	Criteria were vague and based on unfounded theoretical assumptions.
II	Attempt to use atheoretical concepts that would fit with the ICD system.	Criteria were actually based on psychoanalytic concepts. Criteria were too loose.
III	Precise rating criteria and definitions for each disorder.	Criteria were incompletely specified.
III-R	Further refinement of diagnostic criteria.	Became outdated with collection of new research evidence on the disorders.
IV	Incorporation of current research evidence on validity and reliability of diagnoses.	

FOCUSING ON RESEARCH

1. Efficacy research takes place under experimental conditions, usually in university-based clinics where therapists are carefully selected, trained, and monitored. Patients with multiple problems are usually excluded. Effectiveness studies are conducted in the "field" (in real-world therapy settings), where clients are not assigned to random groups, for fixed durations, and are not treated according to a predetermined script.

2. Efficacy studies do not take into account real-world situations. Clients' diagnoses often do not fit neatly into one clearly delineated category, which can be treated with a predetermined script. Efficacy studies don't take into account one of the main reasons therapy is successful (when it is), the client-therapist relationship.

3. Probably both. Efficacy studies have a place because they are conducted under experimental conditions. But I would also want to know about real-life experiences from effectiveness studies.

4. ESTs are empirically supported treatments, those which have supportive research findings. Chambliss and Ollendick remind us that while ESTs have limitations, the research conclusions have come from multiple groups of reviewers, and ESTs have been found effective with a diverse group of clients.

FROM THE CASE FILES OF DR. SARAH TOBIN: THINKING ABOUT PETER'S CASE

1. Peter reported recent bouts of anxiety, feeling "hyper" and restless. However, he reported depression and suicidal ideation four months prior. Don, Peter's brother, corroborated that Peter had been acting "hyper." Peter's mother reported that Peter's landlord observed "odd" behaviors, such as staying up all night, playing his guitar, writing what Peter said was a "million-dollar recording hit." He sometimes ran from room to room, waking up other boarders, telling them to come watch his genius at work. He spent hours on the phone, trying to contact recording executives. He had spent large sums of money, filled out an application to buy a $50,000 car, and looked at expensive homes, as if he could afford these purchases. He hung out in bars in the evening, and, after spending

48 hours with a woman, he asked her to marry him. She did not show up at city hall to get the marriage license, infuriating Peter.

2. Dr. Tobin observed Peter to be "hyper," edgy, irritable, and annoyed when she questioned him. She noticed an air of bravado. He was loud and demanding, but had some endearing qualities. She believed that, beneath the brave front, he was terrified by his experiences since his wife had left him.

3. Dr. Tobin diagnosed Peter with mania, a mood disorder.

4. Dr. Tobin hospitalized Peter voluntarily and ordered lithium to stabilize his mood, individual therapy, family therapy (with his mother and brother) and group therapy with others who were suffering with the same disorder. He stayed in the hospital for 14 days, during which his mania resolved and he ate and slept with more normalcy. He had six sessions of individual therapy, which went well, as did his family therapy. Peter refused to participate in group therapy, saying he had nothing in common with the "psychos" in the group. After discharge, Peter continued individual therapy once every other week for six months, continued to take lithium, and had no return of manic symptoms. He applied for a job in a bank that offered educational benefits. After six months Peter stopped talking the lithium, saying he didn't need it any longer. He cut back his sessions with Dr. Tobin to once a month. After five months of no medication, he exhibited manic symptoms again and Dr. Tobin convinced him to resume his medication. He continued to see Dr. Tobin once monthly for another year, and then therapy was terminated. Since termination of therapy, Peter contacts Dr. Tobin yearly and he reports that "all is well."

5. It appears that Peter's treatment was effective. Though he is not "cured," the symptoms are controlled by lithium. He got and maintained a job and reports periodically to Dr. Tobin that things are going well.

REVIEW AT A GLANCE

1. half
2. 25
3. 15
4. psychiatry
5. psychology
6. social work
7. nursing
8. family
9. *Diagnostic and Statistical Manual of Mental Disorders, 4th Ed (DSM-IV-TR)*
10. reliability
11. validity
12. medical
13. diseases
14. axes
15. clinical disorders
16. personality disorders and mental retardation
17. general medical conditions
18. psychosocial and environmental problems
19. Global Assessment of Functioning (GAF) scale
20. decision tree
21. differential diagnoses
22. principle diagnosis
23. case formulation
24. treatment
25. immediate management
26. short-term goals
27. long-term goals
28. treatment site
29. psychiatric hospital
30. outpatient service
31. halfway house
32. day treatment program
33. modality
34. individual psychotherapy
35. couple or family therapy
36. group therapy
37. milieu therapy
38. quality of the client-clinician relationship

MULTIPLE CHOICE

1. The answer is (c). None of the others are licensed medical doctors.
2. The answer is (a). (b) and (c) apply to test instruments and (d) is a measurement used in some types of assessment.
3. The answer is (b). (a) and (c) don't involve loss of contact with reality, and (d) is a collection of symptoms associated with a certain disorder.
4. The answer is (c). (a) and (b) concern mental health disorders, and (d) is the axis where psychosocial and environmental stressors are listed.
5. The answer is (d). The others are not residential facilities.
6. The answer is (a). Recent studies have been criticized due to their lack of attention to sociocultural differences
7. The answer is (c). (a) involves the likelihood of someone having a disorder, (b) is a collection of symptoms

that may be present in a disorder, and (d) is involved in certain types of assessment.

8. The answer is (b). (a) is what a clinician does when he or she names the disorder; and (c) is the likelihood of recovery from a disorder.
9. The answer is (d). The *DSM* is atheoretical, so (a), (b), and (c) are incorrect.
10. The answer is (b). (a) and (d) are coded on Axis I. (c) would be coded on Axis III, or on Axis I if it affected mental functioning
11. The answer is (a). (c) refers to an assessment issue; (b) is not a term used by diagnosticians; and (d) is related to diagnoses under the *DSM*.
12. The answer is (d). (a) involves relating the symptoms to a known disorder; (b) is the prospect of recovery; and (c) is how the *DSM* categorizes disorder.
13. The answer is (b). None of the others are residential treatment facilities.
14. The answer is (b). Due to his behavior he cannot get to work on time each day. (a) is not a criterion for a mental disorder. It is not a culturally normal behavior (c) and there is no evidence that the behavior causes him any harm (d).
15. The answer is (c). All the other answers are involved after diagnosis.
16. The answer is (d). They are working on long-standing patterns, not immediate (a) and (c) short-term issues; would have resolved at the beginning of treatment.
17. The answer is (c). There are no more asylums (d); (a) and (b) are not outpatient venues.
18. The answer is (a). (d) is where people may live after release from a hospital; (b) is an abbreviation for Community Health Centers; and (c) no longer exist.
19. The answer is (c). (a) and (b) involve other models of psychotherapy; and (d) is a type of psychotherapy involving several clients.
20. The answer is (d). (a), (b), and (c) may be included in (d), which is an integrative approach.

CHAPTER 3
ASSESSMENT

CHAPTER AT A GLANCE

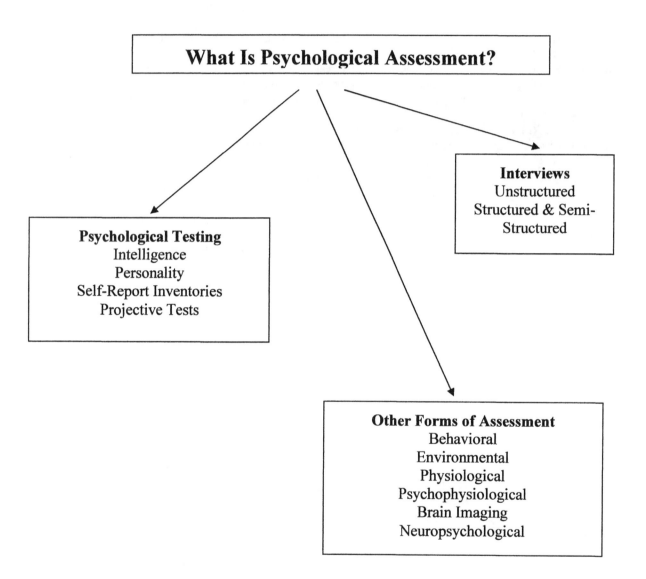

What Is Psychological Assessment?

Psychological Testing
Intelligence
Personality
Self-Report Inventories
Projective Tests

Interviews
Unstructured
Structured & Semi-
Structured

Other Forms of Assessment
Behavioral
Environmental
Physiological
Psychophysiological
Brain Imaging
Neuropsychological

10. _____ False belief that one's thoughts are being transmitted to others who hear these thoughts.
11. _____ Abnormally slow bodily movements and lethargy.
12. _____ False belief that other people are putting thoughts into one's mind.

Identifying Tests

Write in the blank next to each test the aspect (or aspects) of functioning it is designed to assess:

I = intelligence   D = diagnosis   H = physical
P = personality   S = psychophysiological N = neuropsychological

a. ____ Stanford-Binet   g. ____ TAT   m ____ GSR
b. ____ Luria-Nebraska   h. ____ EEG   n. ____ WISC-III
c. ____ Rorschach   i. ____ NEO-PI-R   o. ____ PET scan
d. ____ IPDE   j. ____ Halstead-Reitan p. ____ MRI (or NMR)
e. ____ WAIS-R   k. ____ CAT scan   q. ____ MCMI-IIII
f. ____ MMPI-2   l. ____ Bender-Gestalt

Letter Find Puzzle

The following letters are all used in the definitions below. As you fill in each definition, cross out the letters that you have used until none are left:

```
O I Y S E R T S O A
N T D O M C O Y P N
N I I S I S S C U I
E T O T D L O E P F
O T B N A L M H C N
A A S T A H F L S
C O S A N C S U E H
I S C E M E N T U A
R S O S L I R N T O
I P C A N I O I S E
```

1. Unwanted repetitive thoughts or images that persist in an individual's consciousness.   _ _ _ _ _ _ _ _ _
2. Deeply entrenched false beliefs that are not consistent with an individual's level of intelligence or cultural background.   _ _ _ _ _ _ _ _ _
3. Repetitive behaviors that seem to have no purpose and that are performed in response to a person's uncontrollable urges or according to a ritualistic set of rules.   _ _ _ _ _ _ _ _ _ _ _
4. Disturbance of motor behavior in a psychotic disorder that does not have a physiological cause.   _ _ _ _ _ _ _ _ _

5. Term referring to the "measurement of the mind" and used in describing standards for good psychological tests. _____

6. False perception that does not correspond to any objective stimuli in a person's surroundings. _____

7. Adjective used to describe sadness, used in abnormal psychology to apply to a person's sad mood. _____

8. An individual's awareness of time, place, and personal identity. _____

9. Outward expression of an emotion. _____

10. Process of evaluating an individual's psychological or physical status. _____

Short Answer

1. For each of the methods of assessment listed in the chart, describe the procedures involved in the assessment, the advantages of this method, and its disadvantages.

Assessment method	Assessment procedure	Advantages	Disadvantages
Unstructured interview			
Structured Interview			
Individual intelligence testing			
Self-report clinical inventory			
Projective test			
Behavioral self-report			
Behavioral observation			

2. Answer each of the following questions about the MMPI/MMPI-2:

a. How does the MMPI-2 determine whether a test-taker has falsified responses, been excessively defensive, or been careless in responding?

_____
_____
_____

b. Identify the MMPI-2 scale that is intended to reflect each of the following personality or diagnostic attributes:

_____1. Feelings of unhappiness and low self-esteem
_____2. Asocial and delinquent behaviors
_____3. Elevated mood
_____4. Obsessions, compulsions, and unrealistic fears
_____5. Bodily reactions to stress, denial of psychological problems
_____6. Preoccupation with physical problems and illness
_____7. Bizarre thinking and behavior

c. What was the original intent of the MMPI?
_____
_____

d. How were the MMPI scales developed?
_____
_____

e. Specify three criticisms of the MMPI that the authors of MMPI-2 attempted to address.
_____
_____

f. What five improvements were made in the MMPI-2 in response to criticisms of the MMPI?
_____
_____

3. Identify the types of reliability or validity described in each of the following items:

a. The extent to which two raters agree on how to score a particular response.
b. How closely test scores correspond to related measures at the same point in time.
c. The degree to which items on a test are correlated with each other.
d. How well test scores on one occasion predict performance on other measures at a later occasion.
e. General term applying to how closely test scores correspond to other measures with which they are expected to relate.
f. The extent to which scores taken on the same test at two different occasions relate to each other.
g. How closely a test measures a body of knowledge that it is designed to assess.
h. The degree to which a test measures a concept based on a theoretically derived attribute.

a. _____
b. _____
c. _____
d. _____
e. _____
f. _____
g. _____
h. _____

4. The following questions relate to the concept and measurement of intelligence:

a. How was the "IQ," or intelligence quotient, originally calculated in the Stanford-Binet measurement of intelligence?

_____

_____

b. How does the "deviation IQ" used in the Wechsler scales differ from the original Stanford-Binet IQ?

_____

_____

c. What three forms of IQ are derived from the Wechsler measures of intelligence?

_____

_____

d. What types of measures are used to assess the three forms of IQ?

_____

_____

e. How do clinicians interpret scores on the Wechsler IQ scales?

_____

_____

Focusing on Research

Answer the following questions about the Research Focus entitled "Is Intelligence Destiny?"

1. What is the main thesis of *The Bell Curve* by Herrnstein and Murray?

_____

_____

2. What racial differences in intelligence are proposed by Herrnstein and Murray?

_____

_____

3. List three criticisms that have been made of the Herrnstein and Murray position.

_____

_____

From the Case Files of Dr. Sarah Tobin: Thinking About Ben's Case

Answer the following questions about the case of Ben Robsham.

1. What was Ben's reason for wanting to see Dr. Tobin?

_____

_____

2. What behaviors did Dr. Tobin observe in Ben?

_____

_____

3. Summarize what Dr. Tobin believed to be Ben's history relevant to his current mental state.

_____

_____

4. What evaluation procedures did Dr. Tobin use to assess Ben?

_____
_____
_____

5. According to Dr. Tobin, what psychological disturbances was Ben manifesting?

_____
_____
_____

6. What treatment recommendations and referrals did Dr. Tobin make for Ben?

_____
_____
_____

Social Context

Answer these questions about "Psychological Testing of Diverse Populations."

1. Summarize the general questions raised about the validity of using common psychological tests with people from diverse cultural and ethnic backgrounds.

_____
_____
_____

2. Describe SOMPA and explain how it might be better suited than a standard IQ test (such as the WISC-III) for cognitive assessments of minority children.

_____
_____
_____

3. Briefly state the debate about the validity of using standard personality tests for assessment of ethnic minorities.

_____
_____
_____

4. How is the TEMAS test different from the TAT and other traditional personality instruments and how might its use contribute to a more valid assessment of adaptive and maladaptive aspects of the personalities of minority children living in urban areas?

_____
_____
_____

5. What are some ways a test administrator can reduce potential adverse impact of psychological tests on diverse populations?

_____
_____
_____

Assessing Family Environment: The Global Family Environment Scale

1. Why is it important that mental professionals in various countries generally agree on family environment ratings:

_____

_____

2. How is Adequate Family Environment defined? Give an example of what Poor, Very Poor and Extremely Poor environments would be like.

_____

_____

Review at a Glance

Test your knowledge by completing the blank spaces with terms from the chapter. If you need a hint, consult the chapter summary.

(1)_____ is a procedure in which a clinician evaluates a person in terms of (2) _____, (3) _____, and (4) _____ factors that influence an individual's functioning. Clinicians who undertake assessments have many different goals, depending on the needs of the client. These include (5) _____, (6) _____, and (7) _____. Some assessment tools focus on (8) _____, others assess (9) _____, and others are oriented toward (10) _____.

The (11) _____ is the most commonly used assessment tool for developing an understanding of a client's current problems, past history, and future aspiration. An (12) _____ interview is a series of open-ended questions. The (13) _____ interview consists of a standardized series of questions.

Clinicians use the (14) _____ to assess a client's behavior and functioning in several areas. They include (15)_____, (16)_____, (17)_____, (18)_____, (19)_____, (20)_____, (21)_____, (22)_____, (23)_____, and (24)_____.

Scorable information about psychological functioning is collected through the use of (25) _____, developed and administered according to psychometric principles such as (26) _____, (27) _____, and (28) _____. Information about an individual's cognitive function is obtained through (29) _____. Useful data about a person's thoughts, behaviors, and emotions are obtained through (30) _____, such as the (31) _____, a self-report clinical inventory, and the (32) _____, a projective technique.

Other forms of assessment include behavioral assessment that measures a person's (33) _____, environmental assessments that provide information about (34) _____, physiological techniques, which measure (35) _____, and brain imaging techniques, such as

(36) _____. A commonly used neuropsychological assessment is the (37)

_____.

Based upon information from a wide variety of sources, clinicians formulate an understanding of the (38) _____, (39) _____, and (40) _____ factors that may be important in assessing and treating the client.

Multiple Choice

1. Dr. Tobin uses an assessment approach with open-ended questions on reasons for coming to therapy, health symptoms, family background, and life history. This is called a(n)
   a. unstructured interview.
   b. structured interview.
   c. mental status examination.
   d. self-report.

2. A researcher studying depression has each research assistant ask the same questions in the same order to each subject. This is called a(n)
   a. unstructured interview.
   b. structured interview.
   c. mental status examination.
   d. personal history interview.

3. What term would a clinician use to describe a client's understanding and awareness of self and world?
   a. judgment
   b. reactivity
   c. self-monitoring
   d. insight

4. Edward believes that his thoughts, feelings, and behaviors are controlled by the window fan in his room. This symptom is called a
   a. delusion of control.
   b. visual hallucinations.
   c. somatic delusion.
   d. delusion of nihilism.

5. Marnie cannot rid her mind of thoughts of contamination. This symptom is called a(n)
   a. compulsion.
   b. obsession.
   c. thought disorder.
   d. delusion.

6. An assessment method in which the individual rates family or social context is known as a(n)
   a. behavioral observation.
   b. *in vivo* observation.
   c. behavioral interview.
   d. environmental assessment.

7. A psychologist constructs a measure of "optimism" intended to correlate with other characteristics reflective of optimism. This is known as _____ validity.
   a. construct
   b. criterion
   c. concurrent
   d. content

8. A school psychologist measuring the IQ of a fourth-grade boy could administer the
   a. WAIS-R.
   b. WISC-III.
   c. WPPSI-R.
   d. WBIS.

9. The "mental age" approach used with the Stanford-Binet was abandoned because
   a. scores were hard to determine for adults.
   b. the term "mental" has a negative meaning.
   c. it did not yield Performance and Verbal IQ.
   d. it was based on a deviation measure of IQ.

10. A clinician concerned about whether or not a client has faked responses on the *MMPI-2* would pay careful attention to
    a. the number of items answered.
    b. the elevation of the clinical scales.
    c. the elevation of the validity scales.
    d. the elevation of the reliability scales.

11. Which test used ambiguous pictures that evoked unusual and idiosyncratic responses in the textbook case of Ben Robsham?
    a. Rorschach
    b. MCMI-III
    c. MMPI-2
    d. SCL-90-R

12. A technique for studying the brain involving a computerized combination of X-rays is called
    a. computerized axial tomography.
    b. magnetic resonance imaging.
    c. nuclear magnetic resonance.
    d. positron emission tomography.

13. A disturbance in thought or the use of language is referred to as a(n)
    a. thought disorder.
    b. illusion.
    c. delusion.
    d. obsession.

14. Dispute over the issue of using personality tests in personnel selection has focused on whether
    a. test scores should relate to brain scans.
    b. minority applicants may be unfairly judged.
    c. there are no ethical guidelines for their use.
    d. personality tests have no validity.

15. Inconsistency between the person's expression of emotion and the content of speech is called
    a. mobility of mood.
    b. perseveration.
    c. inappropriateness of affect.
    d. flat affect.

16. A good psychological test is one that follows standardized procedures for scoring and
    a. diagnosis.
    b. classification.
    c. organization.
    d. administration.

17. What kind of psychological test yields information about cognitive deficits and strengths?
    a. projective test
    b. intelligence test
    c. behavioral assessment
    d. self-report questionnaire

18. Which of the following is the most commonly administered self-report inventory?
    a. Wechsler Adult Intelligence Scale-R
    b. *Diagnostic and Statistical Manual of Mental Disorders*
    c. Minnesota Multiphasic Personality Inventory
    d. Rorschach Inkblot Test

19. Dr. Schwartz asks his client to keep a tally of the number of times per hour he says negative things to his wife. This assessment technique is
    a. behavioral interviewing.
    b. self-actualization keying.
    c. self-monitoring.
    d. behavioral observation.

20. Which of the following is an assessment measure specifically designed for use with individuals from diverse cultural and ethnic backgrounds?
    a. NEO-PI-R
    b. SCORS
    c. WISC-III
    d. SOMPA

21. Which of the following is NOT one of the areas of functioning assessed by the mental status examination?
    a. behavior
    b. content of thought
    c. socioeconomic status
    d. motivation

22. Donnie's dad has asked him to turn the radio off, and Donnie responds by repeating, "Radio, radio, radio, radio." This repetition is an example of
    a. habituation.
    b. clanging.
    c. echolalia.
    d. confabulation.

23. All of the Wechsler IQ tests have two sets of scales—one yields a verbal IQ and the other yields
    a. Mathematical IQ.
    b. Cognitive IQ.
    c. Performance IQ.
    d. Psychomotor IQ.

24. Pat's therapist is showing him various inkblots and asking them to tell her what he sees in each. Pat's therapist is administering the
    a. Rorschach.
    b. TAT.
    c. MMPI-2.
    d. BCT.

25. Which of the following is the psychological test specifically designed to assess neurological functioning?
    a. the Wechsler Intelligence Scale for Children
    b. the Electroenchephalogram
    c. Thematic Apperception Test
    d. the Minnesota Multiphasic Personality Inventory.

Answers

MATCHING

1.	g	9.	n
2.	j	10.	e
3.	k	11.	b
4.	l	12.	f
5.	c	13.	d
6.	m	14.	i
7.	o	15.	h
8.	a		

IDENTIFYING SYMPTOMS

1. hyperactivity
2. delusion of grandeur
3. magical thinking
4. dysphoric mood
5. delusion of poverty
6. psychomotor agitation
7. normal or euthymic mood
8. delusion of persecution
9. euphoric mood
10. thought broadcasting
11. psychomotor retardation
12. thought insertion

IDENTIFYING TESTS

1. a. I
   b. N
   c. P
   d. D + P
   e. I
   f. D + P
   g. P
   h. S
   i. P
   j. N
   k. H
   l. N
   m. S
   n. I
   o. H
   p. H
   q. D + P

LETTER FIND PUZZLE

1. OBSESSIONS
2. DELUSIONS
3. COMPULSIONS
4. CATATONIA
5. PSYCHOMETRICS
6. HALLUCINATION
7. DYSPHORIC
8. ORIENTATION
9. AFFECT
10. ASSESSMENT

SHORT ANSWER

1.

Assessment method	Assessment procedure	Advantages	Disadvantages
Unstructured interview	Open-ended questions about personal and family history, symptoms, and reasons for seeking treatment.	Flexibility allows interviewer to adapt questions and questioning style to client's responses.	Variation from interviewer to interviewer in nature of questions.; skill and experience are necessary.
Structured Interview	Highly structured set of questions with predetermined wording and order.	No extensive knowledge of interviewing techniques required. Standardized ratings based on research criteria can be obtained.	No flexibility or adaptation to the situation at hand.
Individual intelligence testing	Standardized questions that tap different verbal and nonverbal abilities.	Rich qualitative information about the client's thought processes and judgment.	Cultural bias; lack of clear support for validity of test scores in terms of relation to behaviors in everyday life.
Self-report clinical inventory	Standardized questions with fixed response categories that the test-taker completes on his or her own.	Are "objective" in that scoring does not require judgment by clinician; can be given to large numbers of people.	Questions are "subjective" in that they often have a theoretical basis, and interpretation of scores can be affected by clinician's biases.
Projective test	The test-taker is presented with ambiguous item or task and asked to "project" his or her own meaning onto it.	Assumed to tap unconscious determinants of personality.	Difficulties in establishing reliability and validity.
Behavioral self-report	Behavioral interviews, self-monitoring, and checklist.	Detailed information about symptoms, goals for intervention, and basis for evaluation.	It is difficult for client to report certain behaviors. Detailed background information is hard to obtain. . Limited to truthfulness of client and to client's willingness to share.
Behavioral observation	*In vivo* or analog observations of the target behavior(s).	Avoids the problem of clients attempting to present themselves in a favorable light on self-report measures.	Observations affect the people whose behavior is being observed.

2. a. There are three validity scales that ascertain how defensive the test-taker was and whether the individual may have been careless, confused, or intentionally lying.

   b. (1) Depression (2); (2) Psychopathic deviate (4); (3) Hypomania (9); (4) Psychasthenia (7); (5) Hysteria (3); (6) Hypochondriasis (1); (7) Schizophrenia (8).

   c. To provide an assessment device that was efficient to administer and score, and that could be used for the purposes of objectively arriving at diagnoses of psychological disorders (a "cookbook").

d. The procedure of "empirical criterion keying" was used. Items developed by the test authors were administered to psychiatric patients and to nonpsychiatric hospital patients and others. Items on which these groups differed and were sensitive to psychiatric diagnosis were included in the final scales of the MMPI.

e. The comparison group of "normals" did not reflect the population diversity of the United States. Many items were outdated or offensive by current standards. The psychometric data in support of the MMPI were only moderate.

f. A more representative sample was used to collect data on normal individuals as well as on psychiatric patients. The items were brought up-to-date. Subcultural biases were eliminated. More subtle validity scales were included. Additional personality assessment scales were included.

3. a. interjudge reliability
   b. concurrent validity
   c. internal consistency
   d. predictive validity
   e. criterion validity
   f. test-retest reliability
   g. content validity
   h. construct validity

4. a. IQ was originally calculated as the ratio of "mental age" to "chronological age."
   b. The deviation IQ is based on conversion of a person's actual test score to a score that reflects how high or low the score compares with the scores of others in that person's age and gender group.
   c. Verbal IQ; Performance IQ; Full Scale IQ
   d. Verbal IQ: vocabulary, factual knowledge, short-term memory, and verbal reasoning
      Performance IQ: psychomotor abilities, nonverbal reasoning, and ability to learn new relationships
      Full Scale IQ: the total of scores on both the Verbal and Performance IQ measures
   e. Scores on the Wechsler scales are interpreted by clinicians by referring to published guidelines and by formulating a picture of the client's cognitive strengths and weaknesses on the basis of how the test-taker responded to particular items and the test situation in general. The interpretation must also take into account a person's background, especially when that person's background does not match those on whom the test was standardized.

FOCUSING ON RESEARCH

1. Intelligence is a heritable trait that predicts and possibly causes a variety of social outcomes, including social attainment or failure of the individual as well as problems for society as a whole.
2. Higher overall IQs for Asians compared with those for Whites and Blacks; higher IQs for Whites compared with those for Blacks.
3. There is considerable evidence for environmental contributions to intelligence.
   Intelligence may be a multifaceted trait, and tests of intelligence do not take all abilities into account.
   The definition of distinct races is difficult to make.

FROM THE CASE FILES OF DR. SARAH TOBIN: THINKING ABOUT BEN'S CASE

1. Ben said he wanted to find out about psychological testing.
2. Dr. Tobin observed Ben to be sitting in a corner of the room, staring at the floor, muttering or humming to himself. Although it was a warm day, he had on a wool hat that covered his hair and ears and he had on black leather sports gloves. His voice sounded fearful. Dr. Tobin believed that Ben was experiencing emotional instability and was feeling needy and frightened. Ben reported that police officers had been following him, since he collided with a police car while riding his bike. He was fearful of being prosecuted by the police. He said he wore the hat and gloves to cover up his identifying characteristics in case "someone is trying to find you." But then he laughed at himself, and said he was just kidding.
3. He spent his time in solitary hobbies and had no close friends. His family system was dysfunctional. He said that his mother was a "nut case," who had been in psychiatric hospitals at least twice. Dr. Tobin believed that her behavior and history suggested that she was a schizophrenic. Ben said that his teachers commented about his failure to maintain eye contact with people. He said he found teachers' questions sometimes hard to understand, but teachers thought he was being a "wise guy." After the collision between his bike and a police car, Ben started feeling frightened of police and believed that they were looking for him to arrest him. He worried that his phone was tapped, his mail read, and his food treated with truth serum. He also believed that "Nazi police," sent by the local police, were trailing him.

4. Diagnostic interview, WAIS-III, MMPI-2, Rorschach, TAT, and evaluation by neurologist that included an MRI.
5. Delusional thinking, hallucinations, and extreme anxiety.
6. Referral for psychiatric consultation, recommended evaluation for antipsychotic medication, and long-term psychotherapy to help him develop more adaptive behaviors.

SOCIAL CONTEXT

1. Some experts contend that test content is biased in favor of white, middle-class American culture and values, and that minorities get lower scores than Whites not because they are less intelligent or have more psychological disorders but because the assessment instruments are flawed.
2. SOMPA is a cognitive assessment along three dimensions, medical, social, and pluralistic, that takes into account cultural and linguistic differences of minority children. Assessment items take into account the child's culture and how it differs from dominant Anglo-American culture. SOMPA seems to be suited for predicting academic placement and achievement, but some question its validity for assessing cognitive abilities.
3. It is suggested that some objective personality measures, such as the MMPI, have items that are inapplicable to different ethnic groups. The TAT, a commonly used projective assessment, contains no depictions of minority members. These criticisms question the validity of these tests for minority populations when the content is tied to the dominant culture.
4. TEMAS was designed specifically for Hispanic and African-American children and adolescents as an alternative to traditional personality instruments such as the TAT. It consists of 23 pictures depicting minority children in ambiguous interpersonal situations, which children are asked to interpret. For instance, one picture could be interpreted as an act of stealing or helping behavior. Responses to the ambiguous depictions provide data about adaptive and maladaptive aspects of personality.
5. A test administrator might provide an orientation suggestion to assure that test takers are familiar with the general content of the test. Study materials can also be provided. Recommendations can be made on the best strategies to use while taking a test, such as how to pace yourself or whether or not to guess at items you are not sure of.

ASSESSING FAMILY ENVIRONMENT: THE GLOBAL FAMILY ENVIRONMENT SCALE

1. We live in an increasingly globalized community. It is important that clinicians from different countries agree on key family environment variables and do so without very much training in how to the Scale.
2. An adequate family environment is stable, secure, and nurturing for the child. Care, affection, and discipline are consistently given, and the expectations on the child's behavior are reasonable. In a Poor environment there might be some abuse, poor supervision, frequent changes of residence, or hostile custody battles. In a Very Poor environment there could be cruel discipline, short-lived parent figures, and severe parental conflict. In an Extremely Poor environment things are so bad the child might be made a ward of the state, or put in an institution or into foster care.

REVIEW AT A GLANCE

1. Assessment
2. psychological
3. physical
4. social
5. determining a person's intellectual capacity
6. predicting a person's appropriateness for a job
7. evaluating competence to stand trial
8. brain structure and functioning
9. personality
10. intellectual functioning
11. clinical interview
12. unstructured
13. structured
14. mental status examination
15. appearance and behavior
16. orientation
17. thought content
18. thinking style and language
19. affect and mood
20. perceptual experiences
21. sense of self
22. motivation
23. cognitive functioning
24. insight and judgment
25. psychological testing
26. validity
27. reliability

28. standardization
29. intelligence tests
30. personality tests
31. MMPI-2
32. Rorschach or TAT
33. behavior
34. family environment or other dimension that influences behavior
35. bodily function and structure
36. EEG, CAT scan, and MRI
37. Halstead-Reitan Neuropsychological Test Battery
38. biological
39. psychological
40. sociocultural

MULTIPLE CHOICE

1. The answer is (a). (b) does not involve open-ended questions; (c) does not involve assessment of reasons for therapy, and background; and (d) involves a written questions which the client answers.
2. The answer is (b). (a) is incorrect (see answer to number 1); (c) is incorrect (see answer to number 1); and there is no assessment procedure known as (d).
3. The answer is (d). (a) is a decision-making process; (b) is a response to something; and (c) is a client's awareness of his or her own behavior.
4. The answer is (a). (b) involves seeing things for which there is no physical basis; (c) and (d) are not recognized symptoms.
5. The answer is (b). (a) involves an act; and (d) is a form of disordered thinking
6. The answer is (d). (a) and (b) involve observing a behavior in the client; (c) involves asking the client questions about behavior.
7. The answer is (a). Criterion (b) validity refers to how test scores relate to some other benchmark. Concurrent (c) validity measures how well the test scores relate to other measures taken at the same time. Content validity is how well the test reflects the information it is designed to tap.
8. The answer is (b). The other answers are not IQ assessment scales for children.
9. The answer is (a). The Stanford-Binet defined IQ as the ratio between "mental age" and chronological age. Since 16 was the highest mental age defined for this test, IQ could not be calculated for adults.
10. The answer is (c). The other answers have nothing to do with determining a client's faking.
11. The answer is (a). The other answers do not involve projective tests that are analyzed for idiosyncratic responses.
12. The answer is (a). The other answers do not involve X-ray-type procedures.
13. The answer is (a). (b) involves an unrealistic belief about something that itself is based in reality; (c) is a thought that is not based in reality; and (d) is a repetitive, intrusive thought.
14. The answer is (b). There is no way yet to measure (a); (c) and (d) are false statements.
15. The answer is (c). (a) involves shifts in mood; (b) involves incessantly talking about one topic; and (d) indicates a lack of emotional expression.
16. The answer is (d). The other answers are not involved in the administration and scoring of assessment instruments.
17. The answer is (b). The other processes do not assess cognitive deficits and strengths.
18. The answer is (c). (a) and (d) are not self-administered; (b) is not an assessment instrument, but a diagnostic manual.
19. The answer is (c). (a) and (d) involve therapist questioning and observation; (b) is not a recognized assessment procedure.
20. The answer is (d). (a), (b), and (c) are not, as such, designed for use with diverse populations.
21. The answer is (c). (a), (b), and (d) are assessed by using the mental status examination.
22. The answer is (c). (a) is not related to language; (d) involves fabricating information and (b) involves making up or using words that have similar sounds.
23. The answer is (c). (a), (b), and (d) are not IQ measures.
24. The answer is (a). (b), (c), and (d) do not utilize inkblots.
25. The answer is (c). (a), (b), and (d) do not assess neurological functioning.

CHAPTER 4
THEORETICAL PERSPECTIVES

CHAPTER AT A GLANCE

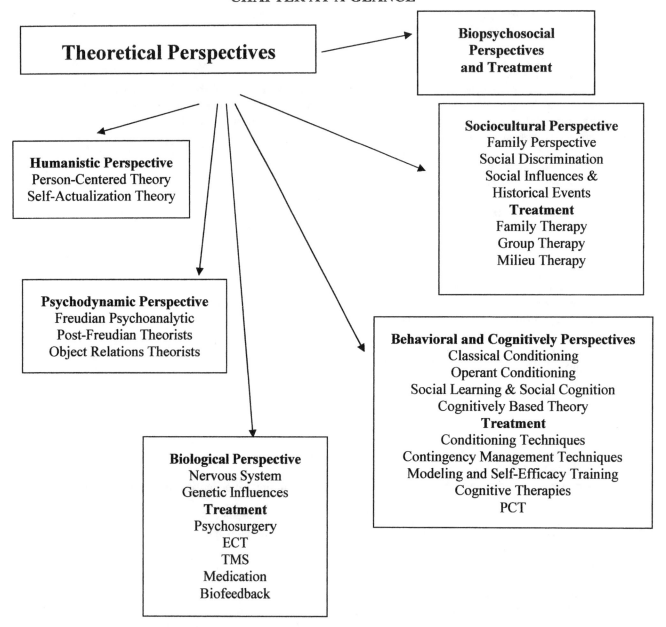

Theoretical Perspectives

Biopsychosocial
Perspectives
and Treatment

Humanistic Perspective
Person-Centered Theory
Self-Actualization Theory

Sociocultural Perspective
Family Perspective
Social Discrimination
Social Influences &
Historical Events
Treatment
Family Therapy
Group Therapy
Milieu Therapy

Psychodynamic Perspective
Freudian Psychoanalytic
Post-Freudian Theorists
Object Relations Theorists

Behavioral and Cognitively Perspectives
Classical Conditioning
Operant Conditioning
Social Learning & Social Cognition
Cognitively Based Theory
Treatment
Conditioning Techniques
Contingency Management Techniques
Modeling and Self-Efficacy Training
Cognitive Therapies
PCT

Biological Perspective
Nervous System
Genetic Influences
Treatment
Psychosurgery
ECT
TMS
Medication
Biofeedback

Learning Objectives

1.0   The Purpose of Theoretical Perspectives in Abnormal Psychology
    1.1   Describe the purpose of theories as the basis for understanding and treating abnormal behavior.

2.0   Psychodynamic Perspective
    2.1   Describe the main concepts of Freud's theory, including the structure of personality, psychodynamics, defense mechanisms, stages of psychosexual development, and Freud's place in history.
    2.2   Describe the theories of other psychodynamic theorists, including Jung, Adler, Horney, Erikson, and the object relations theorists, such as Winnicott and Mahler.
    2.3   Explain the essential features of Freudian psychoanalysis and differentiate this form of therapy from other psychodynamic treatments.
    2.4   Describe the criticisms of Freud's theory.
    2.5   Discuss the research on the role of psychosocial factors and attachment in early personality development, and the growth of new therapeutic models.

3.0   Humanistic Perspective
    3.1   Explain the main concepts of the person-centered theory of Rogers.
    3.2   Outline the main features of Maslow's self-actualization theory.
    3.3   Describe treatment based on the humanistic perspective.
    3.4   Indicate how humanistic theories have contributed to education, industry, and the provision of psychotherapy.

4.0   Sociocultural Perspectives
    4.1   Explain the family systems perspective approach to understanding and treating psychological disorders.
    4.2   Distinguish between the intergenerational, structural, strategic, and experiential approaches to understanding how families and systems can contribute to the development of mental illness.
    4.3   Explain how experiencing gender, race, or age discrimination can cause psychological problems.
    4.4   Describe how general societal forces and historical events can impact on psychological functioning.
    4.5   Outline the methods of family therapy.
    4.6   Describe the methods of group therapy and milieu therapy.
    4.7   Evaluate the contributions of the sociocultural perspective to understanding and treating psychological disorders.

5.0   Behavioral and Cognitively Based Perspectives
    5.1   Explain how principles of classical conditioning have been applied to analysis of the causes of psychological disorder.
    5.2   Distinguish operant conditioning from classical conditioning and show how the principle of reinforcement can be applied to understanding the development of symptoms.
    5.3   Describe the social learning and social cognitive approaches to psychological disorder, including the more recent focus of this approach on self-efficacy.
    5.4   Indicate how cognitively based theories account for psychological disorders, and how faulty cognitions are seen as the cause of emotional distress.
    5.5   Differentiate the behavioral forms of treatment including conditioning techniques such as counterconditioning and desensitization, assertiveness training, contingency management, modeling, and self-efficacy training.
    5.6   Describe the general methods of the cognitive therapies, including cognitive restructuring and PCT.

5.7   Describe the evidence in support of the effectiveness of behavioral and cognitively based approaches to understanding and treating psychological disorders.

6.0   Biological Perspective

6.1   Outline the structure and functions within the central nervous system, the neuron and synapse, neurotransmitters, the structures within the brain, and the autonomic nervous system.

6.2   Describe the role of the endocrine system in behavior, including the effect of hormones.

6.3   Explain basic concepts in genetics, such as genes, chromosomes, genotype, and phenotype.

6.4   Indicate the major models of genetic transmission of inherited traits and diseases as well as the diathesis-stress model.

6.5   Outline the forms of biologically-based therapies, including psychosurgery, ECT, TMS, medication, and biofeedback.

6.6   Evaluate the contributions of the biological perspective, including the search for genetic causes, to understanding and treating mental disorders.

7.0   Biopsychosocial Perspectives on Theories and Treatments: An Integrative Approach

7.1   Explain how integrative models of psychotherapy put together the concepts and methods of the major perspectives in abnormal psychology.

8.0   Chapter Boxes

8.1   Discuss some of the major factors in the case of William Styron.

Matching

Put the letter from the right-hand column corresponding to the correct match in the blank next to each item in the left-hand column.

1. ___ The ego's logical and rational style of thinking.

2. ___ Freud's proposed view of the basis of feminist psychology.

3. ___ Method used by psychoanalysts to encourage client's to talk openly about their unconscious thought process.

4. ___ Stage of development in Freud's theory in which the infant experiences hostile urges toward caregivers.

5. ___ What Adler and Horney regarded as the attempt any maladjusted individual to avoid facing the weaknesses of the self.

6. ___ Object relations theorist who emphasized the infant's fantasy life.

7. ___ What Rogers called the optimally adjusted individual.

8. ___ Psychological process in Maslow's theory characterized by lack of gratification.

9. ___ English psychologist who criticized psychoanalysis as ineffective

10. ___ Process in Freud's theory in which the young child feels romantic love toward the opposite sex parent.

11. ___ The id's distorted cognitive representation of the world.

12. ___ Researcher who developed the "Strange Situation" to study attachment processes in infants.

13. ___ According to Rogers, parental communications that cause children to feel they are loved only if certain demands are fulfilled.

14. ___ Interpretation rejected by Freud that the patients with hysteria he treated were victims of incest.

15. ___ According to Mahler, the most important phase of development.

16. ___ The learning of an association between a neutral stimulus and a behavior that usually occurs reflexively.

17. ___ System in the body involved in controlling automatic, involuntary processes necessary for survival.

18. ___ Brain region involved in controlling balance and motor coordination.

19. ___ Part of the neuron that transmits information to the other neurons.

20. ___ Form of behavioral treatment in which a client receives rewards for performing desired behaviors and not for performing undesired behaviors.

21. ___ System in the body containing the brain and spinal cord.

22. ___ Treatment method in family therapy in which a family is instructed to interact in problematic ways.

23. ___ Type of learning in which the individual acquires new behaviors by being reinforced for performing them.

24. ___ Part of the cortex involved in abstract planning and judgment.

25. ___ Area of the neuron that receives neural transmission.

26. ___ Assumptions or personal rules that interfere with an individual's adjustment.

27. ___ Method of therapy in which a person's negative assumptions and ideas are reframed in more positive ways.

28. ___ Point of communication between two or more neurons

29. ___ Unit of inheritance on which genes are located.

30. ___ Chemical substance produced by the endocrine glands.

a. free association
b. Oedipal complex
c. Hans Eysenck
d. primary process thinking
e. fully-functioning person
f. Mary Ainsworth
g. conditions of worth
h. rapprochement
i. secondary process thinking
j. seduction hypothesis
k. oral-aggressive phase
l. penis envy
m. Melanie Klein
n. neurotic excuses
o. deficit need
p. cognitive restructuring
q. operant conditioning
r. central nervous system
s. dysfunctional attitudes
t. synapse
u. classical conditioning
v. paradoxical intention
w. prefrontal cortex
x. synaptic terminal
y. contingency management
z. hormone
aa. dendrite
bb. basal ganglia
cc. autonomic nervous system
dd. chromosome

Identifying Theories

Put the letter corresponding to the theoretical perspective in the blank next to the concept.

F = Freudian psychoanalysis
P = Post-Freudian psychodynamic (Jung, Adler, Horney, and Erikson)
O = Object Relations (Klein, Winnicott, Kohut, Mahler)
H = Humanistic (Rogers and Maslow)
BI = Biological
FS = Family systems
CB = Cognitive-behavioral
BE = Behavioral
SL = Social learning

various models See themselves as integrative

Perspective	Concept
1. _____	Double bind
2. _____	Automatic thought
3. _____	A-B-C model
4. _____	Extinction
5. _____	Concordance rate
6. _____	Vicarious reinforcement
7. _____	Penetrance
8. _____	Shaping
9. _____	Identified patient
10. _____	Reticular formation
11. _____	Generalization
12. _____	Cross-fostering
13. _____	Self-efficacy
14. _____	Heritability
15. _____	Neurosis results from the individual's misguided efforts to live up to the image of the idealized self.
16. _____	Psychological disorder results from defects in the self, created by faulty parenting.
17. _____	Personality continues to develop throughout life in a series of psychosocial "crises."
18. _____	Psychologically healthy people boost their feelings of well-being by their ability to have peak experiences.
19. _____	Fantasized images in infancy of parents as "good" and "bad" form the basis of the later development of the self.
20. _____	Severe psychological disturbance is the result of faulty communication patterns learned in early life.
21. _____	Psychological disorder is the result of id-ego-superego imbalances.
22. _____	The deepest layer of the unconscious mind is made up of archetypal images representing universal human themes.
23. _____	Psychological disturbance results from incongruence between one's self-concept and one's experiences.
24. _____	Unconscious sexual and aggressive impulses provide the fundamental motivation for human behavior.

Mind Boggler Puzzle

Each box contains a term that is defined in the clue below it. The letters of the term are connected to each other in the box, but they may follow any direction. Indicate your answer by drawing a line connecting the letters in the box.

S U G S C I J P N K Q E G E R Y C V E I P X G O W	B C O X F G P N G R H J T Y U A Q O R E T V E C N	C R F H J L A Q W S U C T X M P O E N B Z Y P C Y	Y E X V Q S B I S T C W M N E O Q T H J V I A L P	T R B W E X V A N X I U E F S N E R O C C E K H G
The structure of personality that, according to Freud, contains the conscience and the ego-ideal	Term used by Rogers to describe a psychological state in which an individual's self-concept is consistent with experiences	Psychosexual development stage in late childhood in which sexual urges become relatively unimportant forces in personality	Theory in psychology that emphasizes living each moment to the fullest	Process in psychotherapy in which the client carries over feelings toward parents onto the therapist

Short Answer

1. Match the theorist or researcher with the concept:

Theorist

___ a. Freud
___ b. Jung
___ c. Adler
___ d. Horney
___ e. Erikson
___ f. Winnicott
___ g. Kohut
___ h. Mahler
___ i. Rogers
___ j. Maslow
___ k Watson
___ l. Bandura
___ m. Minuchin
___ n. Ellis
___ o. Wolpe
___ p. Skinner
___ q. Pavlov
___ r. Bowen
___ s. Haley

Concept

1. psychological crisis
2. narcissism
3. hierarchy of needs
4. idealized self
5. person-centered
6. separation-individuation
7. social interest
8. transitional object
9. libido
10. archetypes
11. power relationships within families
12. irrational beliefs
13. intergenerational approach to family perspective
14. counterconditioning
15. classical conditioning
16. conditioned fear
17. self-efficacy
18. operant conditioning
19. enmeshed families

2. For each of the following theorists, summarize his position on the role of early parenting in the healthy development of the self and the development of psychological disorder:

Theorist	Healthy development	Psychological disorder
Kohut		
Mahler		
Rogers		

3. Describe the contributions, criticisms, and type of research associated with each of the following theoretical perspectives:

Perspective	Contributions	Criticisms	Current evaluation
Psychoanalytic			
Psychodynamic (post-Freudian)			
Humanistic			

4. For each of the following theorists, summarize the goals of treatment and approach or approaches used in therapy:

Theorist	Goals of treatment	Approaches in therapy
Freud		
Adler		
Horney		

Theorist	Goals of treatment	Approaches in therapy
Erikson		
Object relations theorists		
Rogers		

5. Describe the main points, criticisms, and current evaluation of each of the following theoretical perspectives:

Perspective	Underlying assumption about the causes of psychological disorder	Current evaluation
Family systems		
Behavioral (conditioning models)		
Social learning		
Cognitive-behavioral		
Biological		

6. For each of the following theoretical perspectives summarize the goal of treatment approaches used in therapy:

Theory	Goals of treatment	Approaches in therapy
Family systems		
Behavioral (conditioning models)		
Social learning		
Cognitive-behavioral		
Biological		

7. The following behaviors are examples of the ego defense mechanisms identified in Freudian theory. In the blank to the left of each example, name the defense mechanism it represents:

a. _____ Asserting that alcohol is not a problem in one's life, even though one drinks heavily.

b. _____ A person is angry with a roommate and intentionally breaks a glass.

c. _____ After being turned down by a prospective dating partner, a person goes to her room and sulks.

d. _____ A student fails a test and falsely attributes the failure to feeling ill.

e. _____ A daughter insists that she "hates" her mother completely after her mother refuses to lend her money.

f. _____ One mentally relives a tragic situation and makes it come out all right.

g. _____ A soccer player talks about her painful knee operation in a detached and impersonal way.

h. _____ A student forgets about the time he made a fool out of himself at a friend's party.

i. _____ A woman is excessively nice to an acquaintance of whom she is acutely jealous.

j. _____ Someone wrongly accuses a person she is attracted to of flirting with her.

8. Write in the blanks the psychosexual stage with which each characteristic is most closely associated:

O = Oral   A = Anal
P = Phallic   G = Genital

___ a. Smoking
___ b. Being unusually tidy
___ c. Failing to establish a stable career
___ d. Being sarcastic
___ e. Having overly sloppy living habits
___ f. Holding extremely harsh standards of moralistic behavior
___ g. Being unable to share in romantic relationships
___ h. Failing to establish a sense of morality

9. Indicate in the blank next to each item which aspect of Maslow's theory it pertains to, using the following codes:

P = peak experiences
H = hierarchy of needs
S = self-actualization

a. ___ The fulfillment of security needs before the fulfillment of self-esteem needs.
b. ___ Feeling a tremendous surge of inner happiness and harmony with the outside world.
c. ___ The need for physical comfort and safety take priority over reading a good book.
d. ___ Feeling that one can accept one's own weaknesses.
e. ___ Liking people without having to approve of what they do.
f. ___ Achieving a strong sense of spiritual fulfillment.
g. ___ Having a sense of purpose or mission in life.
h. ___ Feeling loved enough by others to go on and seek ways to improve one's self-understanding.

10. As a child, Sandy became terrified when she almost fell out of a fast-moving roller coaster. Now, as an adult, Sandy feels panicky when she takes her children to a park or fair where there a roller coaster is present. Apply the terms from the classical conditioning model of Pavlov to Sandy's experience:

Unconditioned stimulus_____
Unconditioned response_____
Conditioned stimulus_____
Conditioned response_____

Bonus Puzzle

This is an "acrostic" puzzle in which the letters in the clues, when rearranged, form a quotation. The clues are common words, and when you put the letter in each clue in the numbered space in the puzzle, the quote will contain Sigmund Freud's perspective on the use of dreams in understanding personality:

___ ___ ___ ___   Sound made by a lion.
1 18 8 6

___ ___ ___ ___ ___   What you do when you say "One, two, three."
17 2 24 19 12

___ ___ ___   Sodium hydroxide (rhymes with "pie").
5 3 14

___ ___ ___ ___   Sound made by an owl.
13 7 23 10

___ ___ ___   The opposite of happy.
25 4 9

___ ___ ___ ___ ___ ___   Son of your aunt and uncle.
21 11 15 20 22 16

| 1 | 2 | 3 | 4 | 5 | | 6 | 7 | 8 | 9 | | 10 | 11 | | 12 | 13 | 14 | | 15 | 16 | 17 | 18 | 19 | 20 | 21 | 22 | 23 | 24 | 25 |

From the Case Files of Dr. Sarah Tobin: Thinking About Kristin's Case

Answer the following questions about the case of Kristin Pierpont.

1. Summarize Kristin's thoughts and feelings that had led to her see Dr. Tobin..

   _____

   _____

2. What was Dr. Tobin's diagnosis of Kristin?

   _____

   _____

3. Identify the theoretical perspectives Dr. Tobin considered in developing her case formulation (for instance, what models did she use to explain Kristin's psychological state?).

   _____

   _____

4. Describe how Dr. Tobin's treatment plan integrated several theoretical models. Be sure to identify the models and their contributions to Kristin's treatment.

   _____

   _____

   _____

5. Referring to the text box on the feminist-relational approach to therapy, explain how this perspective could contribute to understanding and treating Kristin's psychological distress.

   _____

   _____

Social Context

Answer these questions about: "Feminist-Relational Approaches to Therapy."

1. Explain how the feminist-relational perspective differs from the psychodynamic perspective in explaining the causes of psychological problems.

   _____

   _____

2. Describe how a feminist-relational therapist differs from a psychodynamic therapist in terms of goals of treatment.

   _____

   _____

3. Do you think the feminist-relational approach has some value for men? If so, for what types of psychological problems?

   _____

   _____

Review at a Glance

Test your knowledge by completing the blank spaces with terms from the chapter. If you need a hint, consult the chapter summary.

The five major theoretical perspectives that influence the ways in which clinicians and researchers interpret and organize their observations about behavior are (1) _____, (2) _____, (3) _____, (4) _____, and, (5) _____. The (6) _____ approach brings together aspects and techniques of more than one theoretical perspective.

The (7) _____ perspective emphasizes unconscious determinants of behavior, and is derived from the (8) _____ approach of Sigmund Freud. The term (9) _____ is used to describe the processes of interaction among the (10) _____, (11) _____, and the (12) _____. According to this theory, people use (13) _____ to keep unacceptable thoughts, instincts, and feelings out of conscious awareness. Freud proposed that people develop though a series of (14) _____ stages, with each stage focusing on a different sexually excitable zone of the body: (15) _____, (16) _____, (17) _____ and (18) _____. Post-Freudian theorists, such as (19) _____, (20) _____, (21) _____ and (22) _____ departed from Freud's emphasis of sexual and aggressive instincts. (23)_____ theorists, such as (24)_____, (25)_____, (26)_____, and (27)_____, proposed that (28)_____ lie at the core of personality.

Traditional psychodynamic treatment incorporates techniques such as (29) _____, (30) _____, (31) _____, and (32) _____. Newer approaches, based on object relations theory, have adapted the concept of (33) _____ to understanding the ways that individuals relate as adults to significant people in their lives.

The (34) _____ perspective believes that people are motivated to strive for (35) _____ and (36) _____ in life. The person-centered theory proposed by (37) _____, focuses on the uniqueness of each individual and the need to confront honestly the reality of his or her experiences in the world. (38)_____ self-actualization theory focuses on the maximum realization of the individual's potential for (39)_____ growth. In (40) _____ therapy, Rogers recommended that clients treat their clients with (41) _____ and (42) _____, while providing a model of (43) _____ and a (44) _____.

Theorists within the (45) _____ perspective emphasize the ways individuals are influenced by (46) _____, (47) _____, and (48) _____. The four

major approaches to the (49) _____ perspective are: (50) _____, (51)

_____, (52) _____, and (53) _____. Psychological disturbances can

arise as a result of (54) _____, (55) _____, or (56) _____

discrimination. Treatments within the sociocultural perspective depend upon the nature of social forces

contributing to their distress, and include (57) _____, (58) _____, and (59)

_____.

According to the (60) _____ perspective, abnormality is caused by faulty

(61) _____. According to the (62) _____ perspective, abnormality is caused by

(63) _____ processes. Emotional reactions may be acquired through (64) _____

and behaviors through (65) _____. Behavioral therapists believe that clients can acquire new

emotional and behavioral responses by (66) _____ the behavior of others. The (67)

_____ theories of Beck and Ellis emphasize changing (68) _____.

The (69) _____ perspective sees abnormal emotions, behaviors and cognitive

processes as being caused by (70) _____, such as the (71) _____ and

(72) _____ and (73) _____. A person's (74) _____ makeup can

play an important role in determining certain disorders. In trying to assess the relative role of (75)

_____ and (76) _____, researchers have come to accept an interactionist

perspective. Biological treatments usually consist of (77) _____. (78) _____ is an

intervention in which clients learn to control various bodily reactions associated with stress.

In contemporary practice, most clinicians take an (79) _____ approach, combining

different models by means of (80) _____ (81) _____, and (82)

_____.

Multiple Choice

1. Freud's statement that "the child is father to the man" means
   a. early life experiences play a formative role in the development of personality.
   b. children are often more psychologically healthy than adults.
   c. adults can learn a great deal by observing the behavior of children.
   d. resolution of the Oedipal conflict is needed for healthy adult functioning.

2. Id is to ego as
   a. instinct is to conscience.
   b. secondary is to primary process thinking.
   c. pleasure principle is to reality principle.
   d. ego is to superego.

3. As discussed in the Critical Issue on "repressed" memories of early childhood abuse:
   a. memory of early life events is highly accurate and reliable.
   b. adults accused of abuse confess to their behavior when confronted.
   c. children's memories are not necessarily accurate and are subject to distortion.
   d. clinicians agree that such memories should not be discussed in therapy.

4. According to Freudian theory, which behavior would suggest fixation at the anal stage?
   a. compulsive pursuit of gratification.
   b. a drive to "work and love."
   c. hostility and a critical attitude.
   d. rigid over-control and hoarding.

5. Every time that Alyssa enters her therapist's office, she feels anxious and apprehensive, feelings similar to her fearful reactions to her father. Psychodynamic theorists would call this response
   a. transference.
   b. countertransference.
   c. resistance.
   d. a defense mechanism.

6. The Q-sort was used by Carl Rogers to measure
   a. incongruence between actual and ideal self.
   b. incongruence between actual and real self.
   c. degree of an individual's self-actualization.
   d. an individual's capacity for empathy.

7. Which theorist conceptualized a pyramid-like structure called the hierarchy of needs specifying the order in which human needs must be fulfilled?
   a. Mahler
   b. Laing
   c. Maslow
   d. Rogers

8. Existential theorists believe
   a. it is important to appreciate fully each moment as it occurs.
   b. fundamental flaws in human nature cause psychological disorders.
   c. unconscious factors are the basis of human behavior and existence.
   d. human existence represents a continual struggle between good and evil.

9. What is the term for the phase of psychodynamic treatment in which the client is helped to achieve a healthier resolution of earlier childhood issues?
   a. transference
   b. working through
   c. dream analysis
   d. free association

10. Feminist-relational approaches to therapy emphasize which themes?
    a. the need of the client to establish herself independently of her relationships
    b. the client's need to understand her relationships in terms of penis envy
    c. the relationship between the client's physical and psychological symptoms
    d. the client's feelings about significant relationships and connections in her life

11. Which of the following statements best characterizes current thinking regarding the theoretical perspective that should be assumed by a clinician?
    a. Clinicians typically adopt one perspective from which to treat all individuals.
    b. Most clinicians tend to identify with one perspective but borrow from other perspectives when appropriate.
    c. Most clinicians view the psychodynamic perspective as outdated and therefore utilize the humanistic perspective.
    d. Currently, most clinicians are disillusioned by the psychological perspectives and have adopted the medical perspective.

12. When defense mechanisms are used in a rigid or extreme fashion, they become the source of
    a. adjustment.
    b. psychological disorders.
    c. ego strength.
    d. unconscious impulse

13. Each of Freud's psychosexual stages centers around
    a. the mother-infant bond.
    b. one of the body's erogenous zones.
    c. psychosocial crises in childhood.
    d. development of adequate defense mechanisms.

14. Which post-Freudian theorist claimed that each person goes through a life-long set of 8 crises?
    a. Adler
    b. Horney
    c. Erikson
    d. Sullivan

15. George's psychoanalyst is urging him to sit back, relax, and say whatever is on his mind. This technique is known as:
    a. dream analysis.
    b. free association.
    c. client centering.
    d. word association.

16. To counteract the conditions of worth a person experienced in childhood, Rogers believed that clients should be treated with
    a. sympathy.
    b. unconditional positive regard.
    c. courtesy.
    d. dream analysis.

17. The family perspective was developed in the late 1960s within the emerging framework of
    a. humanistic theory.
    b. systems theory.
    c. behavioral theory.
    d. integrative theory.

18. Eduardo's therapist recommends biofeedback for his high blood pressure because this technique
    a. helps a person to learn how to regulate autonomic functions.
    b. teaches a person to learn how to regulate peripheral nervous functions.
    c. incorporates structured techniques for managing diet and exercise.
    d. is an effective adjunct to systematic desensitization.

19. The pattern of interrelationships among members of a family is referred to as
    a. family dynamics.
    b. family structure.
    c. interindividual paradigm.
    d. psychodynamics.

20. _____ conditioning is a learning process in which an individual acquires a set of behaviors through reinforcement.
    a. Respondent
    b. Operant
    c. Classical
    d. Pavlovian

21. Which learning technique have parents and animal trainers known for years that establishes complex behaviors through gradual steps?
    a. discrimination training
    b. classical conditioning
    c. punishment
    d. shaping

22. Ideas so deeply entrenched that an individual is not even aware that they lead to disturbing feelings of unhappiness and discouragement are referred to by Beck as
    a. dysfunctional attitudes.
    b. automatic thoughts.
    c. false cognitions.
    d. irrational beliefs.

23. "I must be liked or loved by virtually every other person I come in contact with, otherwise I am worthless." This statement, in Ellis' terms is an example of a(n)
    a. faulty cognition.
    b. dysfunctional attitude.
    c. irrational belief.
    d. activating experience.

24. Although Karen is an extremely competent and effective administrator who gets along well with her subordinates and is well liked, she still feels as though she is not doing a good job. In Rogers' terms Karen is in a state of
    a. congruence.
    b. alienation.
    c. conflict.
    d. incongruence.

25. "I get so mad at my wife for bothering me while I try to get my office work done at home." Which of the following statements represents, in Rogers' terms, a reflection of the previous comment?
    a. "You really don't mean that; after all you married her so you can't be angry with her."
    b. "It really must anger you when she interrupts."
    c. "You must have some unconscious hostility toward you mother."
    d. "Your work frustrates you."

26. Jeremy continually gets drunk in a smoke-filled bar, where the jukebox always plays loud country music. Eventually, even before he starts drinking in this bar, his speech gets slurred. The slurring of his speech in response to the smoke-filled room and the country music is a(n)
   a. unconditioned response.
   b. conditioned stimulus.
   c. conditioned response.
   d. unconditioned stimulus.

27. Which perspective argues that indirect reinforcement can also affect behavior?
   a. family systems
   b. humanism
   c. psychoanalysis
   d. social learning

28. A form of counterconditioning in which the individual is trained to replace intimidated behaviors with more forceful behaviors is called
   a. systematic sensitization.
   b. contingency management.
   c. rational-emotive therapy.
   d. assertiveness training.

29. Excesses of which neurotransmitter are related to schizophrenia, while diminished amounts are associated with Parkinson's disease?
   a. serotonin
   b. dopamine
   c. GABA
   d. norepinephrine

30. Judy has asthma and is being taught by her therapist how to identify the onset of an attack and what steps to take in order to control her attacks. This form of treatment is known as
   a. relaxation therapy.
   b. self-monitoring therapy.
   c. biofeedback.
   d. ECT.

Answers

MATCHING

1. i	9. c	17. cc	25. aa
2. l	10. b	18. bb	26. s
3. a	11. d	19. x	27. p
4. k	12. f	20. y	28. t
5. n	13. g	21. r	29. dd
6. m	14. j	22. v	30. z
7. e	15. h	23. q	
8. o	16. u	24. w	

IDENTIFYING THEORIES

1. FS	9. FS	17. P (Erikson)
2. CB	10. BI	18. H (Maslow)
3. CB	11. BE	19. O (Klein)
4. BE	12. BI	20. P (Sullivan)
5. BI	13. CB	21. F
6. SL	14. BI	22. P (Jung)
7. BI	15. P	23. H (Rogers)
8. BE	16. O	24. F

MIND BOGGLE PUZZLE

SUPEREGO
CONGRUENCE
LATENCY
EXISTENTIAL
TRANSFERENCE

SHORT ANSWER

1.
a.	9	h.	6	o.	14
b.	10	i.	5	p.	18
c.	7	j.	3	q.	15
d.	4	k.	6	r.	13
e.	1	l.	17	s.	11
f.	8	m.	19		
g.	2	n.	12		

2.

Theorist	Healthy development	Psychological disorder
Kohut	Parents communicate to the child their pride in the child's accomplishments, which helps the child develop a favorable sense of self-esteem.	Child develops a disturbed sense of self as a result of parents who fail to show their pride and approval in the child's activities.
Mahler	Infant develops through phases in which an autonomous self develops; healthy development results when the caregiver establishes an appropriate balance between supporting dependence and independence.	Disturbance in the sense of self results from being raised by a caregiver who fails to provide adequate nurturance or does not support the child's establishment of autonomy.
Rogers	Parents who accept and support the child unconditionally promote healthy self-development and congruence between self and experiences.	When parents establish conditions of worth, the child feels loved only when certain demands are fulfilled. This situation ultimately leads to the development of incongruence.

3.

Perspective	Contributions	Criticisms	Current evaluation
Psychoanalytic	First modern psychological theory. First systematic approach to psychological disorder. First approach to emphasize psychological causes of disturbed behavior. Emphasized importance of the unconscious.	Difficult to test empirically. Difficult to disprove on logical grounds. Negative view of women in idea of penis envy. Freud's rejection of seduction hypothesis may have been motivated by political reasons. Traditional psychoanalysis is ineffective.	Some supportive evidence in experimental studies of unconscious processes. Brief therapy make it possible to evaluate therapeutic interventions in controlled studies. Freud's theory now viewed increasingly in terms of the context in which it was developed.
Psychodynamic (Post-Freudian)	Incorporated into psychological theory the importance of cognitive processes, interpersonal relations, and social factors. Many important ideas introduced by individual theorists. Expanded psychotherapy beyond psychoanalysis.	Many concepts are as difficult to test experimentally. Evidence to support theories biased by the nature of the methods used to collect the evidence.	Large number of research studies have supported the ideas of these theorists, including research on Erikson's theory, Adler, and attachment styles.
Humanistic	More positive view of human behavior than that offered by psychodynamic perspective. Widespread influence of humanistic ideas has occurred throughout psychology.	Methods of therapy rely heavily on self-report, making them inappropriate for certain disorders. Downplays role of the unconscious and may therefore be overly simplistic. Given the nature of disorders which the perspective can explain, there is a narrow range of clients for whom therapy is appropriate.	Maslow's theory not well-supported by research. Applications of Maslow to business and industry not widely supported. Emphasis by Rogers on research using the Q-sort, and factors affecting therapy outcome give the theory an empirical base and support the importance of empathy.

4.

Theory	Goals of treatment	Approaches in therapy
Freud	Bring into conscious awareness the individual's unconscious conflicts.	Free association; Dream analysis; Analysis of transference issues; Interpretation of resistance.
Adler	Help the individual lead a more productive life.	Collaboration between client and therapist to examine client's feelings of inferiority and boost sense of inner confidence.
Horney	Help the individual regain lost connections to the inner self.	Help client explore unrealistic demands imposed by the idealized self's expectations, and instead accept the flawed, but "true" self.
Erikson	Achieve more favorable resolutions of psychosocial crises.	Help client discover factors impeding the individual's successful resolution of the psychosocial crisis.
Object relations theorists	Reverse destructive processes that occurred early in the client's life.	Through good "parenting," the therapist tries to restore the client's sense of self and control over the self's boundaries. Empathy in therapeutic relationship helps client feel appreciated and accepted as individual (Kohut).
Rogers	Help clients discover their inherent goodness. Achieve greater self-understanding.	Provide unconditional positive regard; Use empathy to see client's situation as it appears to the client; Reflection and clarification of client's feelings and thoughts; Provide model of genuineness and willingness to self-disclose.

5.

Perspective	Underlying assumption about the causes of psychological disorder	Current evaluation
Family systems	An individual's disorder is a function of disturbance in the family as a whole.	Importance of family increasingly recognized as an influential determinant of some disorders, but rarely are family problems considered the sole basis of serious psychological disturbance.
Behavioral (conditioning models)	Psychological disorder seen as a set of behavioral responses that are controlled by the environment.	These theories are empirically based and straightforward, but lack in-depth approach to understanding the causes of disorders.
Social learning	Psychological disorder can be acquired through observing the behavior of others.	Has become more focused on thought processes. Important emphasis on the role of expectancies as part of the learning process.
Cognitive-behavioral	Dysfunctional emotions are the result of faulty cognitions about the self and others.	Cognitive-behavioral models address some of the criticisms of behaviorism but are limited in their application to specific aspects of personality and psychological disorder.
Biological	Psychological disorder has biological origins.	Increasing evidence is accumulating in favor of biological causes of certain disorders, but there is recognition of the importance of interactions with environmental causes.

6.

Theory	Goals of treatment	Approaches in therapy
Family systems	To help the client by changing the family system of which the client is a part.	Working with the family as a whole, the therapist attempts to change the dynamics of the family. In some cases, paradoxical interventions may be used.
Behavioral (conditioning models)	Provide corrective learning experiences that reduce the frequency of maladaptive behaviors.	Counterconditioning. Systematic desensitization. Assertiveness training. Contingency management.
Social learning	Help client develop more positive self-expectations.	Modeling. Self-efficacy training.
Cognitive-behavioral	Change the dysfunctional thoughts that produce maladaptive emotions.	Cognitive restructuring. Rational-emotive therapy. Stress inoculation training.
Biological	Alter faulty biological processes.	Electroconvulsive therapy. Biofeedback.

7.
a. denial
b. displacement
c. regression
d. rationalization
e. splitting
f. undoing
g. isolation of affect
h. repression
i. reaction formation
j. projection

8.
a. oral
b. anal
c. genital
d. oral
e. anal
f. phallic
g. genital
h. phallic

9.
a. H
b. P
c. H
d. S
e. S
f. P
g. S
h. H

10.
The experience of almost falling from a fast-moving roller-coaster
fear
the sight of a roller coaster
fear

BONUS PUZZLE
ROAR
COUNT
LYE
HOOT
SAD
COUSIN

FINAL ANSWER: "ROYAL ROAD TO THE UNCONSCIOUS"

FROM THE CASE FILES OF DR. SARAH TOBIN: THINKING ABOUT KRISTIN'S CASE

1. Kristin said she was seeking therapy to deal with feelings of isolation, loneliness, and unrelenting feelings of sadness as a result of her father's suicide a year earlier. She said that the year since his death had been the worst year of her life. She saw herself as a failure because of her low income, lack of any friends, and lack of a boyfriend. She had little contact with her mother, and refused to go out when people asked her to join them. She said she was sad and furious about what her father did.
2. Mood Disorder and Identity Problem.
3. Dr. Tobin used psychodynamic (object relations), cognitive-behavioral, and sociocultural models. Kristin's lack of closeness with her mother early in life made her insecure about other important relationships. She turned to her father for emotional support and affection. She needed to feel good about herself again (humanistic) and she needed to improve her relationship with her mother (family).
4. The foundation of the treatment plan was rooted in object relations (psychodynamic). Dr. Tobin would conduct the therapy with strong positive regard for and acceptance of Kristin (humanistic). One goal of therapy would be for Kristin to alter the way she views herself, her family, and other significant people in the world (cognitive). Family therapy would be designed to explore family issues with her mother and sister (sociocultural).
5. This approach stresses the value of relationships to women. Kristin's disturbance arose with the loss of the parent closest to her. Dr. Tobin realized this and the goals of therapy included improving relationships with others—sister, mother, and friends.

SOCIAL CONTEXT

1. The psychodynamic perspective traditionally focuses on deficits and problems in early development and stresses the need to achieve autonomy and independence. The feminist-relation approach stresses the importance of relationships.
2. The goals of psychodynamic therapy are self-knowledge, autonomy, and independence, which enable the individual to separate from parents or parent-figures. The goals of feminist-relational therapy are to help women develop a sense of self based on their ability to care for themselves in the context of caring for others, stressing connectedness with others rather than independence from others.
3. There is every reason to believe that men value relationships and closeness, too, but the importance of them and the skills to make and maintain relationships do not necessarily come naturally to them (due to gender roles and expectations). Boys are taught when very young that they must be self-sufficient and independent. This puts pressure on them not to "need" anyone but themselves. Many men complain that they don't have close friends and that they have problems relating to women in healthy ways. The feminist-relationship approach would help men who wanted to improve their relationships develop a sense of self in the context of caring for others.

REVIEW AT A GLANCE

1. psychodynamic
2. humanistic
3. sociocultural
4. behavioral-cognitive
5. biological
6. integrative
7. psychodynamic
8. psychoanalytic
9. psychodynamic
10. id
11. ego
12. superego
13. defense mechanisms
14. psychosexual
15. oral
16. anal
17. phallic
18. genital
19. Jung
20. Adler
21. Horney
22. Erikson
23. Object Relations
24. Klein
25. Winnicott
26. Kohut
27. Mahler
28. interpersonal relationships
29. free association

30. dream analysis
31. analysis of transference
32. analysis of resistance
33. infant attachment style
34. humanistic
35. self-fulfillment
36. meaning
37. Carl Rogers
38. Maslow's
39. psychological
40. client-centered
41. unconditional positive regard
42. empathy
43. genuineness
44. a willingness to disclose
45. sociocultural
46. people
47. social institutions
48. social forces
49. family
50. intergenerational
51. structural
52. strategic
53. experiential
54. gender
55. race
56. age

57. family therapy
58. group therapy
59. milieu therapy
60. behavioral
61. learning experiences
62. cognitive
63. maladaptive thought
64. classical conditioning
65. operant conditioning
66. modeling
67. cognitive
68. maladaptive thought patterns
69. biological
70. abnormal bodily functioning
71. brain
72. nervous system
73. endocrine system
74. genetic
75. nature
76. nurture
77. medication
78. Biofeedback
79. integrative
80. technical eclecticism
81. theoretical integration
82. attention to common factors

MULTIPLE CHOICE

1. (a) is correct. (b) and (c) may be true, and (d) is a Freudian theory, but none of these address Freud's quoted statement.
2. (c) is correct. (a) involves the id and the superego; (b) is incorrect since secondary process thinking belongs to the ego, not the id; and (d) is incorrect.
3. (c) is correct. There is no empirical support for (a), (b), and (d).
4. (d) is correct. (a), (b), and (c) are not associated with the anal stage.
5. (a) is correct. (b) involves the feelings a client invokes in the therapist; (c) is a client's reluctance to do the therapeutic work; and (d) is a mechanism to protect the ego.
6. (a) is correct. (b) is incorrect and (c) and (d) have no bearing on the Q-sort assessment.
7. (c) is correct. Mahler (a) was concerned with infant development; Laing (b) was a critic of the diagnostic process; and Rogers (d) was concerned with the humanistic perspective.
8. (a) is correct. (b), (c), and (d) are unrelated to existential theory.
9. (b) is correct. (a), (b), and (c) are also utilized in psychodynamic therapy, but do not relate to resolution of issues.
10. (d) is correct. (a), (b), and (c) are not associated with feminist-relational approaches.
11. (b) is correct. (a), (c), and (d) may be true for some clinicians, but not for the majority.
12. (b) is correct. Defense mechanisms are not associated with (a) and (c), and may arise as a result of (d).
13. (b) is correct. (a) and (d) are issues in Freud's perspective; (c) is associated with Erik Erikson, not Freud.
14. (c) is correct. (a), (b), and (d) did not propose stage theories of development.
15. (b) is correct. Psychoanalysts may sometimes use (a); (c) is not clinical technique; and (d) was used in the early days of clinical work, but it is not generally in use today.
16. (b) is correct. Rogers did not utilize (a) and (d); he would likely express (c) but not as a technique.
17. (b) is correct. (a), (c), and (d) were not related to the development of the family perspective.
18. (a) is correct. (d) may be correct sometimes; (b) cannot be regulated by biofeedback; and (c) has nothing to do with biofeedback.

19. (a) is correct. (b), (c), and (d) are not terms dealing with family interaction.
20. (b) is correct. (a) are not terms for learning processes; (c) and (d) are the same thing and involve reflexive biological responses
21. (d) is correct. (b) involves biological, reflexive responses; (a) involves a form of operant conditioning; and (c) may be used with operant conditioning, but it does not help one learn new behaviors.
22. (b) is correct. (a), (c), and (d), though they may correctly state the idea, are not associated with Beck.
23. (c) is correct. (a), (b), and (d) are not associated with Ellis.
24. (d) is correct. (a) is the opposite of (d); and there is no evidence for (b) or (c).
25. (b) is correct. (a) is a verbal challenge; (c) and (d) are conclusions.
26. (c) is correct. (a) is incorrect, because the response was learned; (b) and (d) are incorrect because Jeremy's drunkenness is not a stimulus, but a response.
27. (d) is correct. (a), (b), and (c) do not concern reinforcement as an aspect of learning.
28. (d) is correct. (a), (b), and (c) do not involve replacement of maladaptive behaviors with more adaptive responses.
29. (b) is correct. (a), (c), and (d) are not associated with Parkinson's disease or schizophrenia as specified, but with other disorders.
30. (c) is correct. (a) may help Judy get over an attack; (b) may help her predict an attack; and (d) is a form of treatment used for severe psychological disorders, not asthma.

CHAPTER 5
ANXIETY DISORDERS

CHAPTER AT A GLANCE

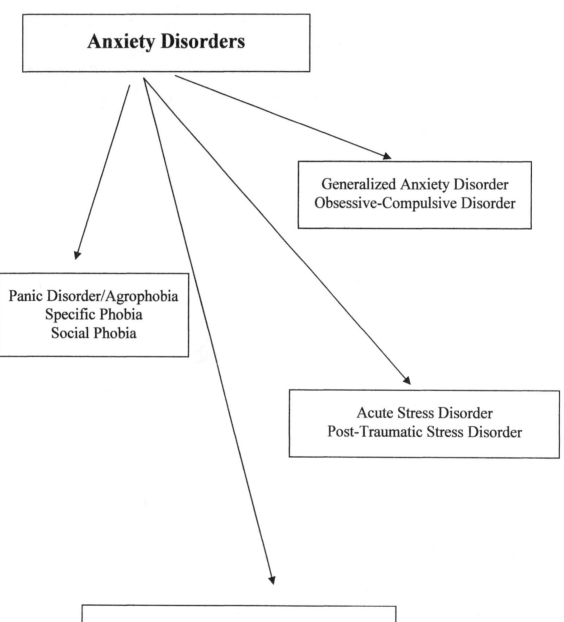

Anxiety Disorders

Generalized Anxiety Disorder
Obsessive-Compulsive Disorder

Panic Disorder/Agrophobia
Specific Phobia
Social Phobia

Acute Stress Disorder
Post-Traumatic Stress Disorder

Theories and Treatments

g. flooding
h. hypervigilance
i. unexpected
j. clomipramine
k. relaxation training

l. obsessive-compulsive disorder
m. fear of fear
n. thought stopping
o. benzodiazepine

Short Answer

1. Describe the role of the following neurotransmitters in anxiety disorders:

Neurotransmitter	Role in panic disorders
Serotonin	
GABA	
Norepinephrine	

2. A behavior therapist is working with a client who has a spider phobia. Describe what treatment approach would be involved in each of the following methods:

Method	Treatment approach
Systematic desensitization	
Graded *in vivo* exposure	
Imaginal flooding	

3. For each of the three approaches used in treating obsessive-compulsive disorder, indicate the mechanism of action and specify a limitation or disadvantage of each approach:

Method	Mechanism of action	Limitation or problem
Behavioral		
Medications		
Psychosurgery		

4. Summarize three forms of evidence used to support the role of biology in obsessive-compulsive disorder:

    _____

    _____

    _____

5. Indicate the main differences between social phobia and panic disorder with agoraphobia:

Social phobia	Panic disorder with agoraphobia

6. Summarize the cognitive-behavioral perspective as applied to each of the following anxiety disorders:

Disorder	Cognitive-behavioral explanation
Panic disorder with agoraphobia	
Specific phobia	
Social phobia	
Generalized anxiety disorder	
Post-traumatic stress disorder	

Acrostic

Fill in the boxes with the term that identifies what is written below the box (or which correctly fits the blank space). When you have completed all of them, place the letter with the number below it in the same numbered space at top of puzzle; when the puzzle is correctly solved, you will have the name of a condition related to anxiety disorders.

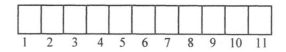

[ ][ ][ ][ ][ ]   [ ][ ][ ][ ][ ][ ]
6

Period of intense fear accompanied by feeling a loss of control.

[ ][ ][ ][ ][ ][ ][ ][ ][ ][ ][ ][ ][ ][ ][ ]
9

Medication most effective in treating symptoms of anxiety.

[ ][ ][ ][ ][ ][ ][ ][ ][ ][ ][ ][ ][ ]
2

Extreme somatic treatment used to treat obsessive-compulsive disorder.

[ ][ ][ ][ ][ ][ ][ ][ ]
4

Systematic desensitization and flooding are behavioral methods that involve _____ to the threatening situation.

[ ][ ][ ][ ][ ][ ][ ][ ][ ]
8

Phase in PTSD in which flashbacks occur.

[ ][ ][ ][ ][ ][ ]
1

Phobia characterized by anxiety over public performance.

[ ][ ][ ][ ][ ][ ][ ]
5

According to one theory, panic attacks are caused by an excess of this chemical in the blood.

[ ][ ][ ][ ][ ][ ]
10

Live presentation of a feared stimulus is used in this form of behavioral therapy.

[ ][ ][ ][ ][ ][ ][ ]
7

_____stopping is used in this form of behavioral therapy.

[ ][ ][ ][ ][ ][ ]
3

The trade name of fluoxetine, a medication that alters serotonin levels in the brain.

[ ][ ][ ][ ][ ][ ][ ][ ][ ]
11

Focusing on Research

Answer the following questions concerning the Research Focus, "The Enduring Effects of Psychological Trauma."

1. What are six possible long-term effects on women of sexual or physical abuse?

    _____

    _____

2. What eight factors are likely to increase the chances that a person exposed to trauma will suffer symptoms of PTSD?

    _____   _____

    _____   _____

    _____   _____

    _____   _____

3. List five types of treatments that are used for PTSD:

    _____

    _____

    _____

    _____

    _____

From the Case Files of Dr. Sarah Tobin: Thinking About Barbara's Case

Answer the following questions about the case of Barbara Wilder.

1. What symptoms did Dr. Tobin observe on first meeting Barbara?

    _____

    _____

2. Describe how Dr. Tobin assessed Barbara.

    _____

    _____

3. Summarize the facts and conclusions that made up Dr. Tobin's formulation of Barbara's case.

    _____

    _____

4. Describe the nature and course of Barbara's treatment.

    _____

    _____

Review at a Glance

Test your knowledge by completing the blank spaces with terms from the chapter. If you need a hint, consult the chapter summary.

Anxiety disorders are characterized by experiences of (1) _____, (2) _____ or _____, (3) _____, (4) _____, and occasionally a (5) _____ or _____.

(6)_____ is characterized by frequent and recurrent (7) _____, intense sensations of fear and physical discomfort. This disorder is often found in association with (8) _____, the fear of being trapped or unable to escape if a panic attack occurs. (9)_____ and (10)_____ perspectives have been particularly useful for understanding and treating this disorder. Treatment based on the cognitive-behavioral perspective involve (11) _____ training and (12) _____ or _____ flooding as ways of breaking the cycle of fear of having a panic attack. The most commonly prescribed medications are (13) _____ and (14) _____ medications.

(15)_____ are irrational fears of particular objects or situations. Cognitive-behaviorists believe that specific phobias are caused by (16) _____ and (17) _____. Cognitive-behavioral treatments include (18) _____, (19) _____, (20) _____, (21) _____, (22) _____, (23) _____, (24) _____, (25) _____, and (26) _____.

A (27) _____ is a fear of being observed by others so as to feel humiliated or embarrassed. Cognitive-behavioral approaches explain this disorder as stemming from an (28) _____. Behavioral treatment methods include (29) _____, (30) _____, and (31)_____.

People with (32) _____ have a number of unrealistic worries that spread to various spheres of life. The cognitive-behavioral approach to this disorder emphasizes the (33) _____ nature of these worries. Treatment is geared toward (34) _____.

In (35) _____, individuals develop (36)_____, thoughts they cannot get rid of, and (37)_____, irresistible and repetitive behaviors. The cognitive-behavioral approach sees these symptoms as the product of a (38) _____ between anxiety and the thoughts and acts, which can temporarily relieve (39)_____. The biological explanation for the disorder suggests that it may be associated with an excess of the neurotransmitter (40)

_____. Treatment with medications such as (41) _____ seems to be effective. Cognitive-behavioral treatment methods include (42) _____ and (43) _____.

In (44)_____, the individual is unable to recover from anxiety associated with a traumatic life event, such as a tragedy, a disaster, an accident, or combat experience. The aftereffects of the traumatic event include (45) _____, (46) _____, and (47) _____ that alternate with (48)_____. A more brief form of the disorder is known as (49) _____. Cognitive-behavioral approaches regard the disorder as a result of (50) _____ thoughts, feelings of (51)_____, (52)_____ from others, and a (53)_____ outlook on life. Treatment includes combinations of covering techniques, such as (54) _____ therapy and (55) _____. (56)_____ techniques include imaginal flooding and (57)_____.

Multiple Choice

1. Which anxiety disorder is most common in young children?
   a. separation anxiety disorder
   b. obsessive-compulsive disorder
   c. generalized anxiety disorder
   d. panic disorder with agoraphobia

2. In people with panic disorder, the association of uncomfortable bodily sensations with memories of the previous panic attack can lead to a full-blown panic attack, a phenomenon known as
   a. unconditioned response.
   b. anticipatory response.
   c. conditioned fear reaction.
   d. prepanic aura.

3. Henri's job involves taking an elevator to the 35th floor, but his claustrophobia is creating serious problems. His therapist vividly describes people trapped in elevators, and asks Henri to imagine the scenes, an approach called
   a. imaginal flooding.
   b. systematic desensitization.
   c. *in vivo* desensitization.
   d. decompensation.

4. What antidepressant medication might be prescribed for obsessive-compulsive disorder?
   a. chlorpromazine
   b. chlorazepam
   c. clozapine
   d. clomipramine

5. Following a traumatic life event, people go through a series of characteristic responses. The initial reaction, involving a sense of alarm and strong emotion, is called the
   a. outcry phase.
   b. denial/intrusion phase.
   c. traumatic phase.
   d. intrusion phase.

6. The surgical treatment used in extreme cases of obsessive-compulsive disorder is known as
   a. cingulotomy.
   b. hyperthyroidism.
   c. uncovering.
   d. lactate infusion.

7. Treatment of Barbara Wilder began in her home, in which she was guided step-by-step through situations that approximated situations that had terrified her in the past, techniques known as
   a. flooding and medication.
   b. hypnosis and age regression.
   c. symptom mastery and cognitive structuring.
   d. *in vivo* techniques and graded exposure.

8. Marlene told her therapist that since her rape she has been terrorized by experiences that seem like hallucinations, similar to those she once had following LSD use. These experiences are called
   a. flashbacks.
   b. intrusions.
   c. delusions.
   d. obsessions.

9. Which neurotransmitter is activated when an individual is placed under stress or in a dangerous situation?
   a. GABA
   b norepinephrine
   c. serotonin
   d. acetylcholine

10. Every time Jonathan sees a spider, he experiences extreme fear and anxiety. Jonathan would be diagnosed as having
    a. generalized anxiety disorder.
    b. aversion disorder.
    c. obsessive-compulsive disorder.
    d. specific phobia.

11. A woman feels that she must scrub her hands for exactly ten minutes after eating any food. This behavior is called
    a. an obsession.
    b. a compulsion.
    c. a delusion.
    d. a specific phobia.

12. What type of panic attack is an essential element of the diagnosis of panic disorder?
    a. situationally bound
    b. situationally predisposed
    c. agoraphobic
    d. unexpected (uncued)

13. Individuals with panic disorder seem hypersensitive to which chemical in the blood?
    a. insulin
    b. norepinephrine
    c. progesterone
    d. lactate

14. The most effective antianxiety medications are called
    a. neuroleptics.
    b. amphetamines.
    c. benzodiazepines.
    d. narcotics.

15. Which behavioral technique is often successful in the treatment of panic disorder with agoraphobia?
    a. lactate therapy
    b. modeling
    c. relaxation training
    d. flooding

16. Which theoretical perspective views the causes of phobias to be based on the individual's faulty inferences and generalizations?
    a. cognitive
    b. humanistic
    c. existential
    d. psychoanalytic

17. The cognitive-behavioral method in which the client is taught not to have anxiety provoking thoughts is called
    a. imaginal flooding.
    b. thought stopping.
    c. graded thinking.
    d. *in vivo* desensitization.

18. A cognitive-behavioral therapist would treat an individual with generalized anxiety disorder by
    a. teaching the client to recognize and change anxiety-producing thoughts.
    b. using free association to illuminate unconscious conflicts.
    c. actively and empathically listening to the client's concerns.
    d. urging the client to develop an enhanced sense of self.

19. Panic disorder in women is associated with what early childhood experience?
    a. parental illness and substance abuse
    b. overachieving school performance
    c. overindulgence by parental figures
    d. supportive family environment

20. In the treatment of PTSD, clinicians may administer medication to control
    a. impulsivity.
    b. appetite disturbance.
    c. high level of sociability.
    d. anxiety, depression, or nightmares.

21. Shelly experiences intense periods of fear and physical discomfort that interfere with her daily living. Shelly may have a(n)
    a. somatoform disorder.
    b. anxiety disorder.
    c. dissociative disorder.
    d. mood disorder.

22. Which of the following statements about the experience of panic attacks in the general population is true?
    a. Many people have had at least one panic attack by the time they reach adulthood.
    b. Many people experience panic attacks more frequently than they think.
    c. Most people have had panic attacks by the time they were ten years old.
    d. Very few individuals in our society have had a panic attack.

23. The fear of being stranded without help available if a panic attack occurs is called
    a. hydrophobia.
    b. simple phobia.
    c. agoraphobia.
    d. social phobia.

24. Wendy encounters test anxiety in Professor Carey's and Professor Burke's classes, but not in Professor Hart's class? Which of the following best characterizes Wendy's panic attacks?
    a. uncued
    b. situation-bound
    c. cued
    d. situationally predisposed

25. According to the cognitive-behavioral perspective, a full-blown panic attack may be triggered even before the appropriate bodily changes have taken place because of the association of certain bodily sensations with
    a. memories of the last panic attack.
    b. unconscious conflicts.
    c. memories of poor attachments in childhood.
    d. increased lactate levels.

26. An irrational and unabating fear of a particular object, activity, or situation is defined as
    a. agoraphobia.
    b. social phobia.
    c. an aversion.
    d. a specific phobia.

27. The behavioral approach to treating phobias, which involves gradually exposing the client to the feared stimulus while the client practices relaxation exercises is called
    a. systematic desensitization.
    b. flooding.
    c. aversive conditioning.
    d. systematic relaxation.

28. Tom, a 50-year-old man, feels anxious most of the time. His symptoms include dizziness, nausea, trembling, and heart palpitations. He is constantly fidgeting and cannot sit still for a minute. Tom would be diagnosed as having
    a. panic disorder.
    b. generalized anxiety disorder.
    c. attention deficit disorder.
    d. hyperactivity.

29. An urge or drive toward action that leads to the performance of repetitive, ritualistic behaviors is called a(an)
    a. habit.
    b. obsession.
    c. compulsion.
    d. delusion.

30. In general, an increased risk of developing PTSD is correlated with
    a. the severity of the trauma.
    b. the individual's genetic predisposition to other psychological disorders.
    c. how rapidly treatment follows.
    d. drug use.

Answers

IDENTIFYING DISORDERS

1. PTSD
2. SoP
3. GAD
4. PD

5. OCD
6. SpP
7. PD (with agoraphobia)
8. GAD

9. OCD
10. SpP
11. SoP
12. PTSD

MATCHING

1. d
2. f
3. i

4. h
5. o
6. b

7. a
8. c
9. e

10. k
11. j
12. n

13. l
14. m
15. g

SHORT ANSWER

1.

Neurotransmitter	Role in panic disorders
Serotonin	Deficiency of serotonin may be involved in panic disorders, as indicated by efficacy of treatment by fluoxetine, which increases availability of serotonin in the brain.
GABA	It is proposed that panic disorder is due to GABA deficiency; neurons in subcortical brain areas involved in panic attacks become more active with less GABA to inhibit them.
Norepinephrine	There is some evidence that panic disorder is caused by heightened levels of norepinephrine when the individual is placed under stress.

2.

Method	Treatment approach
Systematic desensitization	Teaching the client to relax while imagining coming closer and closer to touching a spider.
Graded *in vivo* exposure	Exposing the client in steps to an actual spider.
Imaginal flooding	Instructing the client to imagine touching and holding a spider.
Flooded *in vivo* exposure	Giving the client a spider to touch and hold until the client no longer feels anxiety.

3.

Method	Mechanism of action	Limitation or problem
Behavioral	Thought-stopping to reduce obsessional thinking; exposure to situations that provoke the compulsions or obsessions.	Successful in 75 percent of cases but does not reduce symptoms in the remaining 25 percent who enter treatment.
Medications	Clomipramine (Anafranil) or SSRI May compensate for serotonin deficiencies in certain individuals with the disorder.	Not effective for all individuals with the disorder.
Psychosurgery	Cingulotomy: cutting neuronal tracts between the frontal lobe and a part of the limbic system.	A radical intervention reserved only for clients who are resistant to other treatment methods.

4. There is a higher concordance rate in monozygotic compared to dizygotic twins.
Symptoms of obsessive-compulsive disorder have been observed in people with neurological disorders that affect the basal ganglia.
Brain imaging studies suggest that there is increased metabolic activity in the basal ganglia and frontal lobes.

5.

Social phobia	Panic disorder with agoraphobia
Anxiety is specific to potentially embarrassing contexts in which one's behavior might be observed by others.	The individual fears going out of a safe place due to a concern that a panic attack may strike.
No unusual response to lactate injection.	Lactate injection can provoke the experience of a panic attack.
Equally common in men and women.	More common in women than men.

6.

Disorder	Cognitive-behavioral explanation
Panic disorder with agoraphobia	Distorted cognitions due to negative sensations and belief that panic attacks are unpredictable and uncontrollable.
Specific phobia	Faulty inferences and overgeneralizations.
Social phobia	Focused attention on imagined criticism.
Generalized anxiety disorder	Focus on worries, which leads to a vicious cycle.
Post-traumatic stress disorder	Excessive guilt and self-blame for traumatic events.

ACROSTIC

panic attack	exposure	lactate	Prozac
benzodiazepines	intrusion	*in vivo*	traumatic
psychosurgery	social	thought	

ACROSTIC ANSWER: Agoraphobia

FOCUSING ON RESEARCH

a.
depression
anxiety
substance abuse
sexual dysfunction
dissociation
interpersonal problems

b.
dissociative symptoms
loss of autonomy
stressful life experiences
greater extent of trauma
prior psychological symptoms
demographic factors
childhood exposure to trauma
genetic predisposition

c.
pharmacological
conditioning
improved coping
"uncovering" techniques
"covering" techniques

FROM THE CASE FILES OF DR. SARAH TOBIN: THINKING ABOUT BARBARA'S CASE

1. Barbara was writhing on the floor in what appeared to be a convulsion. She was gasping for breath, and had the appearance of a frightened child. Her body moved rigidly, she shuffled her feet, and she looked worried.
2. Dr. Tobin conducted an unstructured interview about her childhood, adolescence, and adult life to date. Dr. Tobin then referred Barbara to Dr. Herter for a comprehensive behavioral assessment, that included a focused interview, administration of the Body Sensations Questionnaire and Agoraphobia Cognitions Questionnaire, and Barbara's self-monitoring by means of a Panic Attack Record.
3. Barbara's mother and grandmother may have had similar symptoms, leading Dr. Tobin to hypothesize that Barbara had inherited a biological propensity to develop panic attacks. Barbara's relationship with her parents was stressful. Her mother was overcontrolling and her father unreliable and unpredictable. Barbara felt unable to please either parent, and when she left home she felt guilty about leaving her mother. Barbara's early panic attacks were all connected with some kind of emotional conflict—the unresolved conflict about leaving home and separating from a roommate with whom she had formed attachment. Later attacks generalized to all places outside Barbara's apartment.
4. Based upon the referral by Dr. Tobin, Dr. Herter employed behavioral and cognitive-behavioral techniques, including *in vivo* techniques, graded exposure training, cognitive restructuring, and assertiveness training. Dr. Herter began with home-based therapy. Eventually they progressed to a nearby convenience store, then a mall. Barbara learned new ways to think about panic-arousing situations. She also gained some insight into the connection between her interpersonal conflicts and her panic attacks. She stared calling her mother more frequently. Barbara had a relapse when her mother was pressuring her to return home, but she recovered quickly and continued in individual therapy for an additional six months. She eventually overcame her panic attacks and said that she had developed new ways of solving problems related to the possible attacks and her relationship with her mother.

REVIEW AT A GLANCE

1. physiological arousal
2. apprehension or feelings of dread
3. hypervigilance
4. avoidance
5. specific fear or phobia
6. Panic disorder
7. panic attacks
8. agoraphobia
9. Biological
10. cognitive
11. relaxation training
12. *in vivo* or imaginal
13. antianxiety
14. antidepressant
15. Specific phobias
16. previous learning experiences

17. a cycle of negative, maladaptive thoughts
18. flooding
19. systematic desensitization
20. imagery
21. *in vivo* exposure
22. participant modeling
23. cognitive restructuring
24. self-statements
25. thought stopping
26. increasing the sense of self-efficacy
27. social phobia
28. unrealistic fear of criticism
29. *in vivo* exposure
30. cognitive restructuring
31. social skills training
32. generalized anxiety disorder
33. unrealistic
34. breaking the negative cycle of worry
35. obsessive-compulsive disorder
36. obsessions
37. compulsions
38. learned association
39. anxiety
40. serotonin
41. clomipramine or SSRIs
42. exposure
43. thought stopping
44. post-traumatic stress disorder
45. flashbacks
46. nightmares
47. intrusive thoughts
48. denial
49. acute stress disorder
50. negative and maladaptive
51. ineffectiveness
52. isolation
53. pessimistic
54. supportive
55. stress management
56. Uncovering
57. systematic desensitization

MULTIPLE CHOICE

1. (a) is correct. (c) and (d) are not generally seen in young children; (b) may sometimes be manifest in children.
2. (c) is correct. (a) and (b) are not the correct terms for the described behavior; there is no such condition as (d).
3. (a) is correct. (b) is more gradual exposure therapy, and (c) would not involve imagining; and (d) is not associated with phobia therapy.
4. (d) is correct. (a), (b), and (c) are not normally prescribed for obsessive-compulsive disorder.
5. (a) is correct. (c) is the trauma itself; (b) and (d) occur later.
6. (a) is correct. (b) is a condition, not a treatment; (c) and (d) are other types of therapeutic measures.
7. (d) is correct. (a) is not a step-by-step process; (b) and (c) do not fit the described procedures.
8. (a) is correct. (b)) is more gradual exposure therapy,; (c) and (d) involve thoughts, not sensory experiences.
9. (b) is correct. (a), (c), and (d) are not activated by stress.10.(d) is correct. (a), (b), and (c) do not describe specific phobias.
11. (b) is correct. (a) is a thought that gives rise to (b); (c) is a thought that has no basis in reality; and (d) is an irrational fear about something specific.
12. (d) is correct. (a) and (b) arise in certain situations; and (c) is experienced by some who have panic disorders.
13. (d) is correct. (a), (b), and (c) are not known to be involved in panic disorder.14.(c) is correct. (a) is used to treat schizophrenia; (b) is a stimulant; (d) a painkiller.
15. (c) is correct. (a), (b), and (d) are not normally used to treat agoraphobia.
16. (a) is correct. (b), (c), and (d) do not address an individual's thought processes as causes of disorders.
17. (b) is correct. (a) involves imagining; (c) is not a known technique; and (d) involves therapy in a life-like situation.
18. (a) is correct. (b) and (d) are not the main focus of cognitive-behavioral treatment; and (c) is a method used in humanistic therapy.
19. (a) is correct. (b), (c), and (d) are not implicated in women's experiencing of panic disorder.
20. (d) is correct. (a) and (b)do not normally require medication; (c) is not a problem that needs treatment.
21. (b) is correct. (a), (c), and (d) are not associated with fear and physical discomfort.
22. (a) is correct. (b), (c), and (d) are not supported by theory or empirical evidence.
23. (c) is correct. (a) is fear of water; (b) is not a recognized disorder; and (d) involves fear of social situations.
24. (d) is correct. (a) involves a panic attack unassociated with any situation; (b) is incorrect because Wendy does not encounter panic in all test-taking situations; and (c) does not fit the fact pattern described.
25. (a) is correct. (b), (c), and (d) involve perspectives other than cognitive-behavioral.

26. (d) is correct. (a) is a fear of leaving home and being exposed to the threat of panic attacks; (b) is a fear about social settings and situations; and (c) is something unpleasant, not necessarily feared.

27. (a) is correct. (b) is the opposite of (a); (c) would be counter-indicated in treating phobias; and (d) involves relaxation of the body, not exposure to the feared stimulus.

28. (b) is correct. (a) is time-limited; (c) and (d) are children's behavioral disorders, not an adult anxiety disorder.

29. (c) is correct. (a) is not necessarily associated with an urge or drive; (b) is the thought leading to (c); and (d) is an unrealistic thought or idea.

30. (a) is correct. (b), (c), and (d) are not associated with onset of PTSD.

CHAPTER 6
SOMATOFORM DISORDERS, PSYCHOLOGICAL FACTORS AFFECTING MEDICAL CONDITIONS, AND DISSOCIATIVE DISORDERS

CHAPTER AT A GLANCE

SOMATOFORM DISORDERS
Conversion Disorder
Somatization Disorder & Related Conditions
Body Dysmorphic Disorder
Hypochondriasis
Conditions Related to Somatoform Disorders
Theories and Treatment

**PSYCHOLOGICAL FACTORS
AFFECTING MEDICAL CONDITIONS**
Characteristics
Theories and Treatment

DISSOCIATIVE DISORDERS
Dissociative Identity Disorder
Dissociative Amnesia
Dissociative Fugue
Depersonalization Disorder
Theories and Treatment

Learning Objectives

1.0 Somatoform Disorders
    1.1 Describe somatoform disorders as the translation of psychological conflicts into physical symptoms.
    1.2 Indicate the symptoms of conversion disorder.
    1.3 Enumerate the diagnostic features of somatization disorder, and its related conditions.
    1.4 Describe the characteristics of body dysmorphic disorder.
    1.5 Indicate the symptoms used to diagnose hypochondriasis.
    1.6 Discuss the conditions related to the somatoform disorders such as malingering, factitios disorder, and Munchausen's syndrome by proxy.
    1.7 Contrast the theories and treatment of somatoform disorders.

2.0 Psychological Factors Affecting Medical Conditions
    2.1 Explain the basis of the *DSM-IV-TR* category of psychological factors affecting physical conditions.including psychophysiological disorders and sleep disorders.
    2.2 Discuss the theories and treatments of the *DSM-IV-TR* Category of Psychological Factors Affecting Medical Conditions.

3.0 Dissociative Disorders
    3.1 Indicate the symptoms used in the diagnosis of dissociative identity disorder, explanations of this disorder as due to trauma, and the use of hypnotherapy and cognitive-behavioral treatment methods.
    3.2 Describe the symptoms of dissociative amnesia.
    3.3 Enumerate the diagnostic criteria for dissociative fugue.
    3.4 Indicate the symptoms used to diagnose depersonalization disorder.
    3.5 Discuss the role of trauma as a cause of dissociative disorders as well as other theories and treatment of dissociative amnesia, dissociative fugue, and depersonalization disorders.

4.0 Somatoform Disorders, Psychological Factors Affecting Medical Conditions, and Dissociative Disorders: The Perspectives Revisited
    4.1 Describe how varying perspectives enhance our understanding of the causes and treatment of somatoform and dissociative disorders, and psychological factors affecting medical conditions.
    4.2 Identify sociocultural factors that play major roles in causing or aggravating stress-related disorders.

5.0 Chapter Boxes
    5.1 Discuss the case of actress Anne Heche.
    5.2 Discuss Dissociative Identity Disorder and the legal system.

Identifying Disorders

Write the name of the disorder in the blank next to the symptoms listed.

1. _____ Misinterpretation of normal bodily signs as indicators of disease.
2. _____ State of confusion about personal identity accompanied by a flight from home.
3. _____ Translation of psychological conflict into a set of specific physical symptoms.
4. _____ Disturbance in sleep and daytime functioning due to disrupted sleep-wake schedule.

5. _____ Complaints of physical pain that are medically unexplainable.
6. _____ Exaggerated and unrealistic dissatisfaction with a part of one's body.
7. _____ Condition in which an individual repeatedly wakes up suddenly and in a panic from sound sleep.
8. _____ Development of more than one personality state within the same individual.
9. _____ Chronic form of factitious disorder in which the person's life becomes consumed with pursuit of medical care.
10. _____ Chronic difficulty with getting to sleep.
11. _____ Psychological issues that may be expressed through multiple and recurrent physical symptoms.
12. _____ Recurrent and persistent episodes of feeling disconnected from one's own body.
13. _____ Continuous feeling of a need for sleep and never feeling fully rested.
14. _____ Deliberate fabrication of physical or psychological symptoms for an ulterior motive.
15. _____ Inability to remember personal details and experiences not due to demonstrable brain damage.
16. _____ Feigning of symptoms due to an inner need to maintain a sick role.

Matching

Put the letter from the right-hand column corresponding to the correct match in the blank next to each item in the left-hand column.

1. ___ Field that focuses on study of connections among stress, the nervous system, and the immune system.
2. ___ Treatment shown to be effective for dissociative identity disorder.
3. ___ Condition in which individual feigns signs of physical illness for an ulterior motive.
4. ___ Condition in which normal bodily signs are interpreted as symptoms of disease.
5. ___ A fully developed personality in dissociative identity disorder that is separate from the main personality.
6. ___ Disorders in which a person's physical problems are temporarily linked to a stressful event.
7. ___ Disorder in which a person induces symptoms in another who is under the individual's care.
8. ___ The primary personality in dissociative identity disorder
9. ___ A method of coping in which a person reduces stress by trying to feel better about the situation.
10. ___ Personality type characterized by impatience, irritability, competitiveness, and time pressure.

a. psychoneuroimmunology
b. behavioral medicine
c. localized amnesia
d. host
e. masked depression
f. Type C personality
g. malingering
h. hypnotherapy
i. alter
j. emotion-focused coping
k. Type A personality
l. psychophysiological
m. factitious disorder by proxy
n. hypochondriasis
o. problem-focused coping

11.___ Interdisciplinary approach to psychophysiological disorders in which clients are taught to gain control over physical problems.

12.___ Coping style that involves taking action to address the situation.

13.___ Inability to remember events occurring during a specific time period.

14.___ Personality type characterized by suppressed emotions, compliance, and conformity.

15.___ Condition in which a person feeling distressed and unhappy seeks therapy for a physical disorder.

Short Answer

1. List five reasons for the misdiagnosis of dissociative identity disorder:

_____

_____

_____

_____

_____

2. Explain how each of the following contributes to the way an individual responds to stressful situations:

Context	
Internal or personal qualities	
External or situational resources	

3. Specify the type of amnesia that applies to each of the following cases (assume the amnesia applied only to the period or memory loss described):

	A man forgets everything that happened during the month while his wife was dying of cancer.
	A young woman has no recall of events in her past life following her duty in the Persian Gulf war.
	A man forgets the type of car he drove before a hurricane hit his community.
	An incest victim remembers her childhood only through the time when she was abused.

4. Place an "X" next to the term or name that does *not* belong with the others:

a. Motor disturbances
    Localized amnesia
    Sensory disturbances
    Symptoms simulating physical illness

b. Malingering
    Factitious disorder
    Hypochondriasis
    Munchausen syndrome

c. Dissociative identity disorder
    Pain disorder
    Depersonalization disorder
    Dissociative amnesia

d. Briquet
    Charcot
    Janet
    Kluft

e. Primary gain
    Trauma
    Secondary gain
    Unconscious guilt

5. Contrast the relationship between psychological and physical aspects of functioning represented in each of the following disorders:

Disorder	Nature of physical complaint	Presence of organic problem	Theorized role of psychological factors
Conversion disorder			
Somatization disorder			
Pain disorder			
Body dysmorphic disorder			
Hypochondriasis			
Factitious disorder			
Psychophysiological conditions			

6. Answer the following questions regarding the relationship between psychological factors and physical health.

    a. What is the relationship between the terms "psychological factors affecting physical condition" and "psychosomatic illness"?

    _____

    _____

    b. What is the relationship between the terms "psychological factors affecting physical condition" and "psychophysiological disorders"?

    _____

    _____

    c. How is stress thought to lead to the development of physical symptoms?

    _____

    _____

    d. What does research indicate about the effects of emotional expression on a person's ability to recover from stress?

    _____

    _____

    e. What is the explanation of the relationship between the Type C personality and cancer?

    _____

    _____

    f. How is Type A personality thought to be related to heart disease?

    _____

    _____

7. Describe one positive aspect and one negative aspect of primary and secondary gain from the point of view of the individual with a somatoform disorder:

Type of gain	Positive aspect	Negative aspect
Primary		
Secondary		

8. Describe one problem involved in the treatment of somatoform disorder, dissociative identity disorder, and other dissociative disorders:

Disorder	Problem involved in treatment
Somatoform disorder	
Dissociative identity disorder	
Other dissociative disorders	

9. A woman has just been told that her daughter is in trouble at school, an event that she perceives as stressful. Contrast the emotion-focused and problem-focused ways of coping with this stress in terms of the categories below:

Coping method	Example	Possible positive outcome	Possible negative outcome
Emotion-focused			
Problem-focused			

10.
a. Sam exercises for half an hour before he goes to bed, because it is the only chance he has. He drinks coffee continuously throughout the day, with his last cup after dinner. Since his room is fairly small, he does all his studying on his bed. His unpredictable work hours lead Sam to sleep at different times on different days. Lately, Sam has been feeling exhausted and that he has not been able to sleep enough, and is very worried about this. What are Sam's bad sleep habits?

_____

_____

b. What psychological treatments might a clinician recommend for Sam to improve his sleep?

_____

_____

Focusing on Research

Answer the following questions concerning "Social Contest: Dissociative Identity Disorder as a Legal Defense."

1. In what two ways might a defendant use a claim of dissociative identity disorder as a defense in a criminal trial?

_____

_____

2. What assessment instrument helps clinicians detect malingering of multiple personalities?

_____

_____

3. What facts in the client's history and aspects of current functioning might a clinician look for in an effort to distinguish malingering from a dissociative disorder?

_____

_____

From the Case Files of Dr. Sarah Tobin: Thinking About Rose's Case

1. Describe the sequence of events that led to Dr. Tobin's contact with Rose.

_____

_____

2. Discuss how Dr. Tobin assessed Rose.

_____

_____

3. What were the facts and conclusions that made up Dr. Tobin's formulation of Rose's case?

_____

_____

4. Describe the course and outcome of Rose's treatment.

_____

_____

Review at a Glance

Test your knowledge by completing the blank spaces with terms from the chapter. If you need a hint, consult the chapter summary

In somatoform disorders, conditions in which psychological factors affect medical condition, and dissociative disorders, the (1) _____ expresses (2) _____ conflict and (3) _____ in unusual ways. (4)_____ disorders include a variety of conditions in which psychological conflicts become translated into physical problems or complaints that cause (5) _____ or (6)_____ in a person's life. (7)_____ disorder involves the translation of unacceptable drives or troubling conflicts into (8) _____or (9) _____symptoms that suggest some kind of (10)_____ or (11)_____ condition. (12)_____ involves the expression of psychological issues through multiple and recurrent bodily problems that have no basis in physiological dysfunction. In (13)_____, some kind of pain, which causes intense personal distress or impairment, is the predominant focus of the client's medical complaint. People with (14) _____ disorder are preoccupied, almost to the point of being delusional, with the idea that a part of their body is ugly or defective. Individuals with (15) _____ believe or fear that they have a serious illness, when, in fact, they are experiencing normal bodily reactions. (16)_____ and (17)_____ are associated with somatoform disorders. (18)_____ involves deliberately faking the symptoms of physical illness or psychological disorder for an ulterior motive. In (19) _____, people fake symptoms or disorders, not for any particular gain but because of an inner need to maintain a sick role. In (20) _____, a person induces physical symptoms in another person who is under the individual's care. Theorists consider (21) _____ and (22) _____ gain as the basis for the development of somatoform disorders. Somatoform disorders are best viewed as an interplay of (23) _____, (24) _____, (25) _____, and (26) _____. According to the *DSM-IV-TR* diagnostic criteria, the psychological factors that may affect medical conditions include (27) _____, (28) _____, (29) _____, (30) _____, (31) _____, and (32) _____. Researchers and clinicians have focused on the process by which people learn to deal with (33) _____ and have developed sophisticated theories and techniques pertaining to (34) _____. Experts in the field of (35) _____ are finding answers to complex questions regarding the nature of the (36) _____ relationship.

In (37) _____, the person develops more than one self or personality. The *DSM-IV-TR* criteria capture the essence of what many clients report, namely, (38) _____, (39) _____, and (40) _____. In (41) _____, the individual is unable to remember important personal details and experiences, usually associated with traumatic or very stressful events. (42)_____ is a condition in which a person who is confused about personal identity suddenly and unexpectedly travels to another place. In (43) _____, distortions of mind-body perceptions happen repeatedly and without provocation. Experts agree that dissociative disorders commonly arise as a result of (44) _____, usually associated with experiences of childhood (45) _____. Treatment depends on the nature of the dissociative disorder, but the goal is (46) _____ of the fragmented components of the individual's (47)_____ and (48) _____(49)_____ and other therapeutic techniques are commonly used to attain this goal.

Multiple Choice

1. Rose Marston had no motive for feigning illness and truly believed she had a physical disorder. These factors led to the diagnosis of
   a. factitious disorder.
   b. malingering.
   c. somatization disorder.
   d. body dysmorphic disorder.

2. Job stress often causes Ralph's ulcer to flare up. Ralph seems to have a
   a. psychophysiological condition.
   b. somatoform disorder.
   c. factitious disorder.
   d. dissociative disorder.

3. The behavior characterized by being hard driving, competitive, impatient, and is associated with heart disease is called Type
   a. Z pattern.
   b. B pattern.
   c. C pattern.
   d. A pattern.

4. Researchers urge caution before diagnosing a conversion disorder, because as many as half of those diagnosed as having conversion disorder turn out years later to have had
   a. a true physical illness.
   b. a true psychological disorder.
   c. hypochondriacal symptoms.
   d. dissociative symptoms.

5. People with somatization rarely seek out psychotherapy voluntarily because they
   a. lack the financial resources to pay for therapy.
   b. fear that the clinician might detect their motive for feigning illness.
   c. do not consider their physical difficulties to have an emotional cause.
   d. are too embarrassed to talk about their physical problems.

6. Each of the following disorders involves unexplainable medical symptoms *except*
   a. hypochondriasis.
   b. somatization disorder.
   c. somatoform pain disorder.
   d. conversion disorder.

7. Marlene has repeatedly tried to make her 11-month-old son physically ill, so that she can rush him to the emergency room and receive medical attention. Her condition is called
   a. factitious substitution.
   b. Munchausen's by proxy
   c. malingering.
   d. factitious disorder by proxy.

8. Which of the following questions is not part of the Dissociative Disorders Interview Schedule?
   a. Were you physically abused as a child or adolescent?
   b. Do you feel physical pain that lacks a physical basis?
   c. Do you ever speak about yourself as "we" or "us"?
   d. Do you ever feel that there is another person or persons inside you?

9. Disturbances in the amount, quality, or timing of sleep are referred to as
   a. hyposomnias.
   b. nocturnal dysfunctions.
   c. dyssomnias.
   d. parasomnias.

10. People with depersonalization disorder
    a. have more than one personality.
    b. feel as though they are not real.
    c. forget details about personal identity.
    d. fabricate disturbance to get secondary gain.

11. The higher rate of hypertension in African-Americans compared to Whites is thought by researchers to be due to
    a. lower physiological reactivity to stress.
    b. a tendency to express strong emotions.
    c. lower levels of Type A behavior.
    d. patterns of poverty and discrimination.

12. The inability to recall past events from a particular date up to, and including the present time is called
    a. continuous amnesia.
    b. generalized amnesia.
    c. selective amnesia.
    d. psychogenic amnesia.

13. Disorders in which psychological conflicts are translated into physical complaints are the
    a. anxiety disorders.
    b. dissociative disorders.
    c. personality disorders.
    d. somatoform disorders.

14. Legal experts and psychologists have found which reaction to be indicative of a true diagnosis of dissociative identity disorder in forensic cases?
    a. extreme distress and interference of symptoms in daily life
    b. emergence of new personalities during therapy
    c. stereotypical criminal personalities as alters
    d. moderate or little distress over symptoms

15. Mr. Warren has seen many physicians, complaining of difficulty swallowing, chest pain, and blurred vision. Medical examination yields no basis for his claims. Mr. Warren seems to have which somatoform disorder?
    a. factitious disorder
    b. psychalgia
    c. pain disorder
    d. somatization disorder

16. Which somatoform disorder is characterized by dissatisfaction and delusional preoccupation with the idea that some part of the body is ugly or defective?
    a. Briquet's syndrome
    b. psychalgia
    c. body dysmorphic disorder
    d. hypochondriasis

17. A man persistently views his mild headaches as an indication he has a brain tumor despite lack of evidence in support of his claim. This individual may be suffering from
    a. conversion disorder.
    b. psychogenic pain disorder.
    c. somatization disorder.
    d. hypochondriasis.

18. In contrast to individuals with dream anxiety disorder, people with sleep terror disorder
    a. have pleasant dreams that cause them to wake up.
    b. do not recall any dream or any unusual occurrences during the night.
    c. move and walk about in their sleep.
    d. usually experience the terror during REM sleep.

19. The central or core personality in dissociative identity disorder is referred to as the
    a. cardinal personality.
    b. nuclear personality.
    c. alter ego.
    d. host personality.

20. The coping style that involves trying to improve one's feelings about the situation is referred to as
    a. emotion-focused coping.
    b. problem-focused coping.
    c. cognitive coping.
    d. confrontive coping.

21. Disorders involving conditions in which psychological conflicts are translated into physical complaints are the
    a. anxiety disorders.
    b. dissociative disorders.
    c. personality disorders.
    d. somatoform disorders.

22. Connie is relatively unconcerned about the fact that she has suddenly lost all sensation in her left hand. This bizarre lack of concern is referred to as
    a. psychalgia.
    b. hysteria.
    c. la belle indifference.
    d. Briquet's syndrome.

23. If an individual suffering from a somatoform disorder only complains of pain that has no physiological basis, he or she may receive a specific diagnosis of
    a. pain conversion disorder.
    b. psychic neuralgia.
    c. somatoform pain disorder.
    d. hypochondriasis.

24. Which somatoform disorder is characterized by the client's dissatisfaction and delusional preoccupation with the idea that some part of his or her body is ugly or defective?
    a. Briquet's syndrome
    b. psychalgia
    c. body dysmorphic disorder
    d. hypochondriasis

25. The fabrication of physical symptoms for the purpose of gaining material rewards or money is referred to as
    a. malingering.
    b. somaticizing.
    c. masking.
    d. catastrophizing.

26. The avoidance of burdensome responsibilities because one is disabled is a
    a. primary gain.
    b. secondary gain.
    c. positive reinforcement.
    d. avoidance reward.

27. Ralph has an ulcer. More often than not, the stress related to his job as an executive gets so bad that his ulcer flares up. Which of the following best describes his condition?
    a. psychological factor affecting a medical condition.
    b. somatoform disorder.
    c. factitious disorder.
    d. adjustment disorder.

28. In which dissociative disorder does an individual develop more than one self, typically in response to some psychological trauma?
    a. dissociative identity disorder
    b. schizophrenia
    c. schizoid personality disorder
    d. dissociative fugue

29. An overwhelming majority of people who suffer from dissociative identity disorder have experienced
    a. heavy drug and alcohol usage in adolescence.
    b. a sudden schizophrenic break during late adolescence.
    c. a difficult Oedipus complex resolution in the phallic stage.
    d. some form of severe sexual or physical abuse in childhood.

30. A dissociative experience in which the individual experiences alterations of mind-body perception ranging from detachment from one's experiences to the feeling that one has stepped out of one's body is called
    a. a fugue state.
    b. depersonalization.
    c. dissonance.
    d. dissociative amnesia.

Answers

IDENTIFYING DISORDERS

1. Hypochondriasis
2. Dissociative fugue
3. Conversion disorder
4. Circadian rhythm sleep disorder
5. Pain disorder
6. Body dysmorphic disorder
7. Sleep terror disorder
8. Dissociative identity disorder
9. Munchausen's syndrome
10. Primary insomnia
11. Somatization Disorder
12. Depersonalization disorder
13. Primary hypersomnia
14. Malingering
15. Dissociative amnesia
16. Factitious disorder

MATCHING

1. a
2. h
3. g
4. n
5. i
6. l
7. m
8. d
9. j
10. k
11. b
12. o
13. c
14. f
15. e

ANAGRAMS

1. CONVERSION
2. PRIMARY
3. HYPNOSIS
4. FUGUE
5. DYSMORPHIC
6. TRAUMA

Final word = MUNCHAUSEN'S

SHORT ANSWER

1. Dissociative identity disorder is linked to epilepsy, schizophrenia, and somatoform disorder.
   The symptoms of dissociative identity disorder are not consistent over time.
   The individual may try to cover up symptoms.
   Dissociative symptoms may be mixed with mood disturbance or personality disorder.
   The individual may be functioning at a high level and not appear to have a disorder.

2.

Context	What precedes an event can influence its effects; an unexpected stress (such as a loss) may be more stressful than one that follows a long period of preparation.
Internal or personal qualities	Internal or personal qualities such as biological, personality, and cognitive vulnerabilities can influence a person's coping resources.
External or situational resources	External or situational resources such as a social network and material resources can help buffer the impact of a stressful event.

3.
Localized
Generalized
Selective
Continuous

4.
a. Localized amnesia
b. Hypochondriasis
c. Pain disorder
d. Kluft
e. Trauma

5.

Disorder	Nature of physical complaint	Organic Problem	Theorized role of psychological factors
Conversion disorder	Involuntary loss or alteration of bodily functioning.	No	Caused by underlying conflict.
Somatization disorder	Multiple and recurrent bodily symptoms.	No	Caused by underlying conflict.
Pain disorder	Pain.	No	Caused by underlying conflict.
Body dysmorphic disorder	Preoccupied with dissatisfaction over appearance of bodily part.	No	Unrealistic perception of appearance.
Hypochondriasis	Exaggerated concern over normal bodily reactions.	No	Acceptable way for finding help for other problems such as depression.
Factitious disorder	Physical or psychological symptoms are feigned.	No	Desire to be center of attention, nurtured, masochistic wish to experience pain.
Psychophysiological	Asthma, headaches, ulcer.	Yes	Psychological factors can initiate, aggravate, or prolong medical problems.

6.

a. The term "psychological factors affecting physical condition" replaces "psychosomatic" based on evidence that such disorders are not "in the person's head."

b. These conditions include situations when a person's physical symptoms are temporally linked to a stressful event. The simpler term "psychophysiological" has traditionally been used to refer to these conditions.

c. A stressful event can lower resistance to disease. Such an event can also aggravate symptoms of a chronic stress-related disorder. Current explanations propose that stress stimulates and lowers immune activity, leaving the body vulnerable to conditions such as gastrointestinal problems, infection, cancer, allergic reactions, and arthritis.

d. Research by McClelland suggests that the suppression of emotions can lead to harmful physical reactions and research by Pennebaker suggests that it can be physically beneficial to put emotions into words.

e. The Type C personality is a proposed personality type identified in cancer victims who cannot express their negative feelings toward others. This activation may lead to chronic arousal of the sympathetic nervous system and lowered efficiency of the immune system, which is involved in the body's natural protection against cancer.

f. People with a Type A personality are thought to be in a state of heightened activation, leading to high blood pressure and risk of heart and arterial disease.

7.

Type of gain	Positive aspect	Negative aspect
Primary	Avoidance of burdensome responsibilities.	Lost wages.
Secondary	Sympathy and attention from others.	Annoyance and anger from others.

8.

Disorder	Problem involved in treatment
Somatoform disorder	Avoid reinforcing the client's adoption of the sick role, but also provide support so that client accepts psychological treatment.
Dissociative identity disorder	Avoid inadvertent reinforcement of other personalities.
Other dissociative disorders	Avoid provoking a dissociative episode in the client by moving too fast through the uncovering of traumatic memories.

9.

Coping method	Example	Possible positive outcome	Possible negative outcome
Emotion-focused	Try to look at the event in positive terms, such as it will help the daughter "grow as a person."	The mother will feel better about the situation.	The mother will fail to intervene on the daughter's behalf, and she may get into more serious trouble.
Problem-focused	Talk to the daughter's teachers and guidance counselors to get at the root of the problem.	Changes may be implemented that help improve the daughter's behavior.	The mother may feel frustrated if she finds that no one at school can really help.

10.

a.

Exercising before bedtime.

Drinking coffee within six hours of bedtime.

Using his bed for activities other than sleeping.

No regular sleep schedule.
Worrying about his sleep problems.
b.
Simple educational intervention to improve his sleep habits.
Behavioral strategies such as relaxation, biofeedback, and cognitive self-control.
Stress management.

FOCUSING ON RESEARCH

1. They may claim that they are not competent to stand trial or that the disorder precluded them from appreciating and understanding their criminal actions.
2. The Structured Clinical Interview for DSM-IV-TR Dissociative Disorders (SCID-D-R) has been particularly useful in evaluating the severity of dissociative symptoms and in diagnosing dissociative disorders in both psychiatric and legal contexts.
3. Evidence of periods of amnesia, personality change, and other aspects of fragmented experience in the client's current functioning that are interfering in everyday life, as well as evidence that the client suffered extreme abuse in childhood; the malingerer would not show emotional scars or abuse and would find it difficult to maintain a consistent façade of dissociated feelings, thoughts, and memories that he or she could associate with different personality traits.

FROM THE CASE FILES OF DR. SARAH TOBIN: THINKING ABOUT ROSE'S CASE

1. The hospital emergency room physician referred Rose to Dr. Tobin. Rose had gone to the emergency room on 15 occasions in the past year complaining about what seemed to be serious medical problems (vomiting; nausea; chest, back, and joint pain; and neurological symptoms), yet doctors could make no diagnosis.
2. Dr. Tobin conducted an interview and administered the WAIS-III, MMPI-2, TAT, and Rorschach.
3. The most important fact was that Rose had a younger sister who was born with severe abnormalities. Emily got all the attention in the family, until Emily died as a teenager. Rose dropped out of college due to a series of unexplainable illnesses and ailments. She could not keep a job due to incapacitating physical symptoms, and she had recently applied for disability benefits. Rose's physical symptoms began after Emily died, suggesting that Rose identified with her sister and took on her symptoms, in part to punish herself for unconscious guilt about being healthy and to keep her from living up to her potential. Rose's symptoms also gave her parents something to focus on after Emily's death. This kept them from dealing with the dysfunctions in their marriage.
4. Therapy had to address the emotional and psychological problems that were underlying the physical symptoms. Dr. Tobin recommended individual, group, and family therapy. Rose rejected family therapy, saying her father would never agree to it. She stayed in individual therapy for only a few weeks before she stopped, saying she had found a cure for her physical problems. Several months later, she was admitted to the emergency room following a suicide attempt through an overdose of pain medication. She resumed therapy with Dr. Tobin, yet she never seemed to make the connection between her physical problems and the difficulties in her emotional life. After she was involved in a car accident and had several minor operations, she phoned Dr. Tobin and said that she would not be returning to therapy because of her need for intensive medical care and rehabilitation.

REVIEW AT A GLANCE

1. body
2. psychological
3. stressSomatoform
5. distress
6. impairment
7. Conversion
8. bodily motor
9. sensory
10. neurological
11. medical

12. Somatization disorder
13. pain disorder
14. body dysmorphic
15. hypochondriasis
16. Malingering
17. factitious disorders
18. Malingering
19. factitious disorder
20. factitious disorder by proxy
21. primary

22. secondary
23. biological factors
24. learning experiences
25. emotional factors
26. faulty cognitions
27. Axis I disorders
28. psychological symptoms
29. personality traits
30. maladaptive health behaviors
31. stress-related physiological

responses
32. less specific psychological factors
33. emotional experiences
34. coping
35. psychoneuroimmunology
36. mind-body
37. dissociative disorders
38. intense detachment
39. disorganization
40. amnesia
41. dissociative amnesia
42. Dissociative fugue
43. depersonalization disorder
44. intense trauma
45. abuse
46. integration
47. personality
48. cognition
49. Hypnoth

MULTIPLE CHOICE

1. (c) is correct. (a) and (b) involve feigning; (d) concerns body image.
2. (a) is correct. (b), (c), and (d) concern disorders for which there is no physical basis.
3. (d) is correct. (a), (b), and (c) are not associated with the described behaviors.
4. (a) is correct. (b), (c), and (d) would be closely related somatoform disorders.
5. (c) is correct. They are not feigning (b), and there is no reason to think that (a) and (d) are accurate statements.
6. (a) is correct. (b), (c), and (d) involve manifestations of disorders; people with (a) do not normally manifest physical symptoms.
7. (d) is correct. (a) is not a disorder; (b) involves making one's self ill; (c) involves feigning illness.
8. (b) is correct. (a), (c), and (d) are part of the interview schedule.
9. (c) is correct. (a), (b), and (d) are not generally used terms for sleep disorders.
10. (b) is correct. (a), (c), and (d) are not associated with the described behaviors.
11. (d) is correct. Evidence does not support (a), (b), and (c).
12. (a) is correct. (b) is more global; (c) is limited to certain memories; and (d) involves amnesia associated with traumatic experiences.
13. (d) is correct. (a), (b), and (c) do not involve physical complaints.
14. (a) is correct. (b) and (c) would indicate a false diagnosis; (d) is not related to dissociative identity disorder.
15. (d) is correct. (a) involves feigning; (b) is not a disorder; (c) involves pain without physical cause.
16. (c) is correct. (b) is not a disorder; (a) and (d) do not involve body image.
17. (d) is correct. (a) and (c) concern disorders for which there is no physical basis; (b) is not a known disorder.
18. (b) is correct. (a) is not a disorder; (c) may indicate sleepwalking or REM disorder; terrors are not experienced in (d), nightmares are.
19. (d) is correct. (a) and (b) are not accepted psychological terms; (c) refers to a psychodynamic theory.
20. (a) is correct. (b) involves focusing on the situation; (c) and (d) are not terms used for dealing with feelings about situations.
21. (d) is correct. (a), (b), and (c) do not involve physical complaints caused by psychological conflicts.
22. (c) is correct. (a) is not a psychological term; (b) is the former term for conversion disorder; (d) is the former name for somatization disorder.
23. (c) is correct. (a) and (b) are not terms used to describe disorders; (d) involves a fear of having a disorder, but with no apparent symptoms.
24. (c) is correct. (a) is the former term for somatization disorder; (b) is not a term used to refer to disorders; and (d) involves a fear of having a disorder with no apparent symptoms.
25. (a) is correct. (b) and (c) do not describe psychological disorders; (d) describes a cognitive process.
26. (a) is correct. (b) refers to the attention and sympathy one may gain when disable; (c) is a term used in operant conditioning; (d) is not a term used to describe a psychological process.
27. (a) is correct. (b), (c), and (d) involve disorders without a physical basis.
28. (a) is correct. (b) is a psychotic disorder; (c) is a personality disorder; and (d) is an anxiety disorder in which a person may wander away from home and temporarily develop a new identity.
29. (d) is correct. (a), (b), and (c) are not associated with development of dissociative identity disorder.
30. (b) is correct. (a) involves wandering away from one's home; (c) is a cognitive process; and (d) involves a loss of memory

CHAPTER 7
SEXUAL DISORDERS

CHAPTER AT A GLANCE

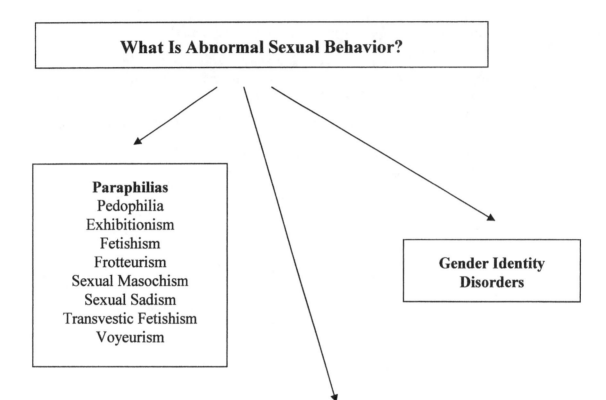

What Is Abnormal Sexual Behavior?

Paraphilias
Pedophilia
Exhibitionism
Fetishism
Frotteurism
Sexual Masochism
Sexual Sadism
Transvestic Fetishism
Voyeurism

Gender Identity Disorders

Sexual Dysfunctions
Hypoactive Sexual Desire
Sexual Aversion Disorder
Female Sexual Arousal Disorder
Male Erectile Disorder
Female Orgasmic Disorder
Male Orgasmic Disorder
Premature Ejaculation
Sexual Pain Disorders

Learning Objectives

1.0   What Is Abnormal Sexual Behavior?
    ~~1.1~~   Discuss the issues involved in defining abnormal sexual behavior.
2.0   Paraphilias
    ~~2.1~~   Explain the characteristic features of paraphilias, including pedophilia, exhibitionism, fetishism, frotteurism, sexual masochism, sexual sadism, transvestic fetishism, and voyeurism.
    2.2   Contrast biological and behavioral explanations of paraphilias.
    2.3   Discuss the treatments of paraphilias.
3.0   Gender Identity Disorders
    3.1   Describe the features that characterize gender identity disorders.
    3.2   Discuss the possible causes of and treatments for gender identity disorders.
4.0   Sexual Dysfunctions
    4.1   Indicate the nature of sexual dysfunctions and their relationship to the human sexual response cycle.
    4.2   Outline the diagnostic criteria for sexual dysfunctions, including hypoactive sexual desire disorder, sexual aversion disorder, female sexual arousal disorder, male erectile disorder, female and male orgasmic disorders, premature ejaculation, and sexual pain disorders.
    4.3   Discuss the roles of biological and psychological factors in the cause and treatment of sexual dysfunctions.
5.0   Sexual Disorders: The Perspectives Revisited
    5.1   Identify the perspectives that have the most promise for understanding and treating sexual disorders.
6.0   Chapter Box
    ~~6.1~~   Discuss some of the key aspects in the case of Richard Berendzen.

Identifying Disorders

Write the name of the sexual disorder in the blank at the left that fits the symptom described at the right.

1.   _____   Intense urges and fantasies involving exposure of genitals to a stranger.
2.   _____   A woman is unable to experience orgasm during sexual activity.
3.   _____   A man cannot attain or maintain an erection during sexual activity.
4.   _____   Strong recurrent sexual attraction to an object.
5.   _____   Recurrent or persistent pain in the genitals during intercourse.
6.   _____   A man reaches orgasm before he wishes during a sexual encounter.
7.   _____   Active dislike of intercourse and other sexual activities.
8.   _____   Sexual gratification derived from rubbing against unsuspecting strangers.
9.   _____   Attraction to sexual situations in which satisfaction is derived from having painful stimulation applied to oneself.
10.   _____   A man has an uncontrollable urge to dress as a woman to achieve sexual gratification.
11.   _____   A woman is convinced that she is a man trapped in the body of woman.
12.   _____   Uncontrollable attraction to children to the point that sexual gratification can be achieved only in their presence or while fantasizing about them.
13.   _____   Attraction to sexual situations in which the individual dominates the partner to the point of causing the partner physical and/or emotional pain.
14.   _____   A man cannot experience orgasm during sexual activity.

Matching

Put the letter from the right-hand column corresponding to the correct match in the blank next to each item in the left-hand column.

1. ___ Behavior or attitudes associated with society's definition of maleness or femaleness.
2. ___ Condition in which a person is solely interested in deriving sexual gratification from a specific part of another person's body.
3. ___ One of the pair of researchers who first studied the human sexual response in the laboratory.
4. ___ Paraphilic behavior in which the individual derives pleasure from dominating or being dominated by a sexual partner.
5. ___ Representation of an individual's sexual fantasies and preferences.
6. ___ Sexual dysfunction in which the man is unable to attain or maintain an erection.
7. ___ Paraphilia in which the individual attains sexual gratification from exposing his genitals to others.
8. ___ Anxiety experienced by a person during sexual intercourse due to preoccupation with his or her performance.
9. ___ Type of pedophilia in which an individual with a normal history of sexual development becomes sexual with a child in certain contexts.
10. ___ Disorder in which the individual feels trapped in the body of the other sex.
11. ___ Individual's attraction to the same and/or other sex.
12. ___ Type of pedophilia in which the individual maintains a continuous interest in children as sexual partners.
13. ___ Sexual dysfunction in which the man reaches orgasm in a sexual encounter before he wishes to.
14. ___ Paraphilia in which a man derives sexual gratification from dressing as a woman.
15. ___ Clinician who developed an integrative approach to treating sexual dysfunctions.

a. preference molester
b. sexual orientation
c. male erectile disorder
d. gender identity disorder
e. Helen Singer Kaplan
f. spectatoring
g. situational molester
h. transvestic fetishism
i. premature ejaculation
j. partialism
k. Virginia Johnson
l. gender role
m. sadomasochism
n. lovemap
o. exhibitionism

Short Answer

1. Indicate the contributions and limitations of Masters and Johnson's research on human sexual functioning:

Contributions	Limitations

2. A client is distressed over the fetish he has about baby's diapers. Describe the following behavioral methods that could be used in treating this client:

Type of method	Description of method
Counterconditioning	
Aversive conditioning	
Covert conditioning	
Orgasmic reconditioning	

3. Describe what is considered "abnormal" about coercing a partner to have sex while tied down, compared with having sex in an exotic place that both partners enjoy:

_____

_____

4. Describe the four subtypes of sexual aggressors identified by Hall and colleagues, and summarize the descriptions and treatments recommended for each type:

Type				
Description				
Treatment				

5. For each of the following somatic treatments for sexual dysfunctions, identify the disorder it is intended to treat, the intended mechanism of action, and problems or disadvantages associated with each:

Somatic treatment	Disorder	Mechanism of action	Problems/ Disadvantages
Administer progesterone			
Surgical implant of penile prosthesis			
Castration			
Sex reassignment surgery			
Hypothalamotomy			

6. Anne is living with her long-term partner, Mary. Describing herself as a "traditional woman," Anne is interested in domestic activities and works as a manicurist. She and Mary have a sexual relationship, and this relationship is consistent with Anne's sense of herself as a woman. Based on this information, answer the following questions:

a. Is Anne's gender role masculine or feminine? Why?

_____

_____

b. Is her gender identity that of a male or female? Why?

_____

_____

c. What is Anne's sexual orientation? Is this consistent with her gender identity? Why or why not?

_____

_____

7. Contrast physical and psychological causes of sexual dysfunctions:

Physical	Psychological

8. Identify which sexual disorder or problem is treated by each of the following methods:

Method of treatment	Sexual disorder or problem
Dilators	
Squeeze technique	
Stop-start technique	

9. Delineate childhood experiences that might result in the development of sexual disorders:

Disorder	Childhood experiences
Paraphilias	
Sexual dysfunctions	
Gender identity disorder	

Word Find

Circle the words defined below in this puzzle.

```
W  L  B  T  M  F  C  I  L  E  C  O  H  C  T
V  O  Y  E  U  R  A  A  P  H  R  K  V  O  B
A  V  U  R  E  O  H  E  R  K  A  O  A  V  Q
R  E  R  E  C  T  I  L  E  R  N  E  R  E  U
E  M  G  C  E  T  N  S  M  A  S  T  E  R  S
S  A  S  F  I  E  U  T  A  D  V  O  D  T  Y
A  P  D  I  E  U  L  O  T  R  E  Y  S  G  E
D  O  I  N  M  R  C  A  U  O  S  A  E  H  Z
I  B  C  I  H  I  D  I  R  C  T  H  C  V  W
S  M  F  A  K  S  D  F  E  T  I  S  H  I  R
T  S  C  R  N  M  B  D  I  S  C  N  I  O  Q
M  O  A  O  A  L  E  W  I  N  E  S  M  N  J
```

1. According to John Money, a disturbance in an individual's _____ is responsible for the development of a paraphilia.
2. In _____ conditioning, the individual learns to associate unpleasant emotional states with the paraphilic behavior.
3. A sexual dysfunction in which a man is unable to achieve or maintain sexual arousal is called male _____ disorder.
4. Researcher who, along with Johnson, brought the study of human sexuality into the laboratory: _____.
5. The paraphilia in which the individual derives sexual pleasure from rubbing his genitals against an unwitting stranger: _____.
6. In the paraphilia called _____ fetishism, a person derives sexual gratification from dressing as a member of the other sex.
7. Individual who derives pleasure from inflicting pain on another person: _____.
8. A person who derives sexual pleasure from secretly watching other people in a nude or partially clothed state, or having sex: _____.
9. In _____ ejaculation, a man is unable to control his orgasmic response until the time during sexual relations that he desires.
10. Strong and recurrent sexual attraction to an object, without which an individual cannot achieve sexual gratification: _____.

Focusing on Research

Answer the following questions about "Research Focus: A Relationship between Pedophilia and a History of Being Sexually Victimized."

1. Summarize the research about the link between child sexual abuse and pedophilia.

   _____
   _____

2. What is the relationship among serious family disturbance, sexual victimization, and victim offending in later life?

   _____
   _____

3. Why is it important to understand the causes of pedophilia?

   _____
   _____

From the Case Files of Dr. Sarah Tobin: Thinking About Shaun's Case

Answer the following questions about the case of Shaun Boyden.

1. Describe Dr. Tobin's impressions of Shaun when she met him for the first time, pursuant to court referral.

   _____
   _____

2. How did Dr. Tobin assess Shaun and what was her diagnosis?

3. What aspects of Shaun's psychosocial history were important for Dr. Tobin's case formulation?

_____

_____

4. Indicate the nature and outcome of Shaun's treatment.

_____

_____

Review at a Glance

Test your knowledge by completing the blank spaces with terms from the chapter. If you need a hint, consult the chapter summary.

Sexual behavior is considered a psychological disorder if it (1) _____ or causes an individual to experience (2) _____ or _____. (3)_____ are disorders, lasting at least (4) _____ months, in which an individual has recurrent, intense sexual arousing fantasies, urges, or behaviors involving (5) _____, (6) _____, or (7) _____. (8)_____ is a disorder in which an adult (9) _____ years of age or over has uncontrollable sexual urges toward (10) _____. In (11) _____, a person has (12) _____ and _____ involving (13) _____. People with (14) _____ are preoccupied with an (15) _____ in order to achieve (16) _____. A (17) _____ has recurrent sexual urges and fantasies of (18) _____ or (19) _____ another person. (20)_____ is a disorder marked by an attraction to achieving sexual gratification by having (21) _____.

(22)_____ involves deriving sexual gratification from activities that (23) _____.

(24)_____ is a disorder in which a man has an uncontrollable urge to (25) _____ (also known as _____) as his primary means of achieving sexual gratification.

(26)_____ is a sexual disorder involving (27) _____. Most paraphilias emerge during (28) _____. Although biological factors play a role in some paraphilias, (29) _____ seem to be central. In most cases, one or more (30) _____ have taken place in childhood involving a (31) _____ that results in a paraphilia. Treatments include (32) _____, (33) _____, and (34) _____ or _____ therapy.

(35)_____ is a condition involving a discrepancy between an individual's (36) _____ and _____ and a sense of inappropriateness about his or her assigned gender. The biological explanation focuses on the effects of (37) _____ that affect (38)

_____. Psychological theories focus on factors such as (39) _____, (40) _____, and the (41) _____. Various factors influence choice of intervention. The most extreme method is (42) _____. (43)_____ involve abnormalities in an individual's sexual (44) _____ and (45) _____. The individual with (46) _____ has an abnormally low level of interest in sexual activity. (47)_____ is characterized by an active dislike and avoidance of genital contact with a sexual partner. A woman with (48) _____ experiences persistent or recurrent inability to attain or maintain normal responses of sexual excitement during sexual activity. (49)_____ involves recurrent partial or complete failure to attain or maintain an erection during sexual activity. (50)_____ is the inability for a woman to achieve orgasm, and (51) _____ involves a man having specific difficulty in the orgasm stage. The man with (52) _____ reaches orgasm in a sexual encounter long before he wishes to. (53)_____, which involve the experience of pain associated with intercourse, are diagnosed as either (54) _____ or (55) _____. (56)_____, which affects both males and females, involves recurrent or persistent (57) _____ before, during, or after sexual intercourse. (58)_____, which affects only females, involves (59) _____ or _____ involuntary spasms of the outer muscles of the vagina. Sexual dysfunctions can be caused by (60) _____ or (61) _____ problems, or by an interaction of both. Treatment of sexual dysfunctions includes (62) _____ and psychological interventions, such as (63) _____, (64) _____, and (65) _____ therapy technique.

Multiple Choice

1. Researchers have noted that this factor may increase the likelihood of sexual offenses in adulthood:
   a. early family conflict and abuse
   b. secure patterns of attachment
   c. highly consistent parenting patterns
   d. lack of physical or sexual abuse

2. Fetishism appears to develop in a way similar to exhibitionism in that
   a. most people with fetishism were sexually abused as children.
   b. early life experiences result in a connection between sexual arousal and the behavior.
   c. brain damage early in life appears to cause certain paraphilias.
   d. these paraphilias are commonly associated with sexual dysfunction.

3. An individual who has recurrent, intense sexual urges and sexually arousing fantasies of rubbing against another person is referred to as a
   a. voyeur.
   b. sadist.
   c. frotteur.
   d. fetishist.

4. Jackson has a normal sexual history; however, following the financial collapse of his company, he sexually molested the young daughter of his business partner. Jackson is considered a
   a. preference molester.
   b. child rapist.
   c. paraphiliac.
   d. situational molester.

5. The most common physiological intervention for treating pedophilia involves
   a. administering the female hormone progesterone.
   b. administering the male hormone testosterone.
   c. psychosurgery called hypothalamotomy.
   d. administering electroconvulsive therapy.

6. Bondage is a term associated with
   a. sexual sadism.
   b. sexual dysfunction.
   c. fetishism.
   d. transvestic fetishism.

7. The phenomenon in which a man derives sexual excitement from the thought or image of himself as having female anatomy, biological characteristics such as menstruation, or the ability to breast-feed is called
   a. transvestic fetishism.
   b. autogynephilia.
   c. inorgasmia.
   d. autoeroticism.

8. Which of the following factors has a positive influence on the postoperative readjustment of people who have had sex reassignment surgery?
   a. the quality of the surgery itself
   b. the individual's marital status
   c. uncertainty about the decision
   d. poor adjustment prior to surgery

9. The term that refers to the degree to which a person is erotically attracted to members of the same or other sex is
   a. sexual orientation.
   b. gender identity.
   c. gender role.
   d. transsexualism.

10. The disorder involving an abnormally low level of interest in sexual activity is called
    a. a paraphilia.
    b. sexual arousal disorder.
    c. hypoactive sexual desire disorder.
    d. orgasmic disorder.

11. A psychopathic sexual murderer is more likely than a murderer with a mood disorder to
    a. leave behind an organized crime scene.
    b. have a history of early sexual abuse.
    c. also have schizoid traits.
    d. also have avoidant personality traits.

12. Dyspareunia is a condition that involves
    a. psychological distress associated with a paraphilia.
    b. depression that accompanies a sexual dysfunction.
    c. involuntary spasms of the outer muscles of the vagina.
    d. pain associated with sexual intercourse.

13. A sexual behavior is considered a psychological disorder if it
    a. is forbidden by state, local, or federal law.
    b. is viewed as unacceptable by society or an individual's culture.
    c. causes harm to others or distress to the individual.
    d. involves unconventional sexual practices.

14. Biological theorists contend that exhibitionistic behavior may be the result of
    a. damage to the ventromedial hypothalamus.
    b. unconscious desires for the parent of the opposite sex.
    c. loss of nervous system control of sexual inhibition.
    d. a cultural emphasis on male dominance.

15. A woman is erotically obsessed with men's ankles to the point of exclusion of all other erotic stimuli. This woman's desires are illustrative of
    a. partialism.
    b. sadism.
    c. frotteurism.
    d. voyeurism.

16. The behavioral intervention geared toward a relearning process in which the individual associates sexual gratification with appropriate stimuli is called
    a. aversion therapy.
    b. orgasmic reconditioning.
    c. cognitive restructuring.
    d. sensate focus.

17. A radical surgical procedure designed to treat individuals with pedophilia involves the destruction of areas of which brain structure?
    a. the pituitary gland
    b the frontal lobe
    c. the hippocampus
    d. the hypothalamus

18. Research regarding the "conversion" of gays and lesbians has shown that these treatments are
    a. are ineffective and may be harmful.
    b. more effective for lesbians than gay men.
    c. successful when used with medication.
    d. recommended by most therapists.

19. An active dislike of intercourse or related sexual activities is the main symptom of which sexual dysfunction?
    a. male erectile disorder
    b. sexual arousal disorder
    c. sexual aversion disorder
    d. hypoactive sexual desire disorder

20. Based on what you have read about Masters and Johnson's technique of sensate focus, in which perspective does this technique seem to be rooted?
    a. psychodynamic
    b. cognitive
    c. humanistic
    d. behavioral

21. Which of the following is the key feature of paraphilias?
    a. The object of desire must be an inanimate object.
    b. They must involve abnormal physiological functioning.
    c. They must be short-term conditions.
    d. There must be a dependence on the sexual target for arousal.

22. Which of the following best describes a preference molester?
    a. an individual who prefers children, especially boys, as his sexual partners
    b. a violent child abuser whose behavior is an expression of hostile sexual drives
    c. an individual who has a normal history of sexual development but is occasionally overcome by pedophilic impulses
    d. a person with normal impulses who occasionally has sex with children

23. Bob has intense recurrent fantasies in which he is walking along the beach and a woman approaches. As she gets near, he unbuttons his pants and exposes his genitals to her. At that instant, she falls madly in love with him and they make love in the sand. Bob occasionally acts out these fantasies, and might be given the diagnosis of
    a. sexual sadism.
    b. exhibitionism.
    c. transvestic fetishism.
    d. frotteurism.

24. Wendy has just purchased a vibrator in order to enhance her sexual arousal when she makes love to her husband. Which of the following statements best describes this situation?
    a. Wendy would be considered a fetishist.
    b. Wendy's husband might be diagnosed with erectile disorder.
    c. Wendy might be diagnosed with hypoactive sexual desire disorder.
    d. Wendy's behavior would not necessarily be considered fetishistic.

25. In which paraphilia does the individual masturbate by rubbing up against an unsuspecting stranger?
    a. pedophilia
    b. voyeurism
    c. transvestic fetishism
    d. frotteurism

26. Which disorder is characterized by a discrepancy between an individual's assigned sex and his or her gender identity?
    a. sexual aversion disorder
    b. hypoactive desire disorder
    c. homosexuality
    d. gender identity disorder

27. Katie is not interested in sexual activity and reports no desire for it, nor does she fantasize about having sex. Katie might be diagnosed as having
    a. hypoactive sexual desire disorder.
    b. sexual arousal disorder.
    c. inhibited female orgasm disorder.
    d. sexual aversion disorder.

28. Dwayne is very interested in sex but his penis remains flaccid despite erotic stimulation. Dwayne has
    a. sexual arousal disorder.
    b. sexual aversion disorder.
    c. male erectile disorder.
    d. inhibited male orgasm disorder.

29. Karen and Mark are being treated for a sexual dysfunction and their therapist is urging them to take turns stimulating each in nonsexual ways for a few weeks. Their therapist is using which of the following methods?
    a. the squeeze technique
    b. the start-stop procedure
    c. systematic resensitization
    d. sensate focus

30. Katasha, 13, likes to wear boy's clothing and play softball. She also likes to wear her hair short and is not interested in makeup or jewelry. Her mother is unnecessarily worried that she might have which of the following disorders?
    a. oppositional defiant disorder
    b. conduct disorder
    c. sexual behavior disorder
    d. gender identity disorder

Answers

IDENTIFYING DISORDERS

1. Exhibitionism
2. Female orgasmic disorder
3. Male erectile disorder
4. Fetishism
5. Dyspareunia
6. Premature ejaculation
7. Sexual aversion disorder
8. Frotteurism
9. Sexual masochism
10. Transvestic fetishism
11. Gender identity disorder
12. Pedophilia
13. Sexual sadism
14. Male orgasmic disorder

MATCHING

1. l
2. j
3. k
4. m
5. n
6. c
7. o
8. f
9. g
10. d
11. b
12. a
13. i
14. h
15. e

SHORT ANSWER

1.

Contributions	Limitations
Dispelled myths about sexuality.	Laboratory setting was artificial.
Provided a scientific basis for understanding sex.	Samples studied were non-random.
Gave a humanistic orientation to sexual functioning.	An implicit sex bias which pathologized women.

2.

Type of method	Description of method
Counterconditioning	Substitute relaxation for arousal in the presence of baby's diapers.
Aversive conditioning	Present a punishing stimulus every time the client touches baby's diapers.
Covert conditioning	Teach the client to imagine being humiliated while masturbating with baby's diapers.
Orgasmic reconditioning	Have the client experience orgasm while in the presence of appropriate sexual stimuli.

3. "Abnormal" sexual behavior involves sexual activity that causes harm to another person or that causes the individual to experience distress. Coercing a partner causes harm to that person; two consenting individuals having sex in an out-of-the-way place is distressing to neither person, even though it may be atypical.

4.

Type	Physiological	Cognitive	Affective	Sexual
Description	Experiences deviant sexual arousal patterns. Victims likely to be male children. Aggressor is less violent than affective or sexual aggressor.	Plans sexual aggression. Victims likely to be acquaintances or relatives. . Aggressor is less violent than affective or sexual aggressor.	Lacks affective control, sexual aggression likely to be impulsive. Depressed aggressors victimize children, and angry aggressors victimize adults.	Long history of personality and adjustment difficulties. Use violence toward victims.
Treatment	Castration, hormonal treatment, and aversion therapy.	Victim empathy training and relapse prevention.	Cognitive therapy for depression or anger.	Cognitive therapy, social skills training, behavior therapy, and prevention in adolescence.

5.

Somatic treatment	Disorder	Mechanism of action	Problems/Disadvantages
Administer progesterone	Pedophilia	Reduce sex drive by reducing testosterone.	Potentially damaging side effects. Lowers ability to respond to appropriate stimuli. May lead to false belief of cure. No change in object of sexual desire.
Surgical implant of penile prothesis	Erectile disorder	Permits erection.	Invasive, possible psychological impact.
Castration	Pedophilia and other dangerous sex offenses	Reduces sex drive by eliminating production of testosterone.	Arousal still possible. Radical intervention. May not eradicate deviant fantasies and wishes.
Sex reassignment surgery	Gender identity disorder	Changes body to be consistent with gender identity.	Results not perfect and hormones still needed. Childbearing potential is lost. Psychological benefits are mixed.
Hypothalamotomy	Pedophilia	Change arousal patterns by targeting source of these patterns in the hypothalamus.	Ethical issues. Destruction of brain tissue can have unintended side effects. May decrease sex drive but not preference for children.

6.
a. Anne's gender role is feminine because she defines herself as "traditional," and has "feminine" interests and a "feminine" job.
b. Her gender identity is that of a female because she views herself as a woman.
c. Her sexual orientation is homosexual. Sexual orientation is independent of gender identity, so there is no basis for an inconsistency between her gender identity as a woman and her sexual orientation as a homosexual.

7.

Physical	Psychological
Illness and disease. Anatomical abnormalities or problems with sex organs. Medications. Drugs.	Misinformation about sex. Spectatoring. Cultural expectations. Relationship problems.

8.

Method of treatment	Sexual disorder or problem
Dilators	Vaginismus
Squeeze technique	Premature ejaculation
Stop-start technique	Premature ejaculation

9.

Disorder	Childhood experiences
Paraphilias	Early associations between sex and inappropriate stimuli.
Sexual dysfunctions	Traumatization and abuse. Learning of negative attitudes toward sexuality.
Gender identity disorder	Reinforcement of cross-gender behaviors.

WORD FIND

1. Lovemap
2. Covert
3. Erectile
4. Masters
5. Frotteurism
6. Transvestite
7. Sadist
8. Voyeur
9. Premature
10. Fetish

FOCUSING ON RESEARCH

1. Some studies have found that many pedophiles were sexually abused as children. Others have observed that the rate of childhood sexual abuse among pedophiles is only slightly higher than that of individuals who commit other sexual offenses. However, men who had been victims of more than one instance of sexual abuse and had also suffered emotional abuse were much more likely to engage in sexual activities with minors, perhaps out of identification with their abusers.
2. Early relationship disturbances with caregivers and sexual abuse within the family are characteristic of the most violent sexual offenders. Because offenders lack adequate models for relationships and for controlling aggressive and sexual impulses, sexual offenses become acceptable outlets for the feelings of isolation, anger, and sexual arousal that these individuals experienced as children.
3. With improved understanding, more effective treatments can be formulated and prevention programs developed in which those at greatest risk of perpetuating the cycle of abuse can be helped before they act on their fantasies and inclinations.

FROM THE CASE FILES OF DR. SARAH TOBIN: THINKING ABOUT SHAUN'S CASE

1. Shaun was 46 years old but he dressed like a teenager, and the harshness of his face made him look a decade older. He appeared uncomfortable and was emotional, weeping as he talking about his sexual urges and the possibility that he might lose his daughters. He denied ever having molested a child before this incident and said his wife knew nothing about his problem.

2. Dr. Tobin administered the WAIS-III, the MMPI-2, the Rorschach, and the TAT, as well as specialized sexual assessment inventories. His IQ was average, his MMPI-2 scales indicated that he was guarded and suspicious, and his Rorschach responses indicated impulsivity and restricted ability to fantasize. This led Dr. Tobin to believe that he could be counted on acting out his immediate impulses without considering the consequences of his actions. His TAT stories contained themes of victimization. The sexual assessment inventories confirmed Shaun's preference for sex with young boys, almost to the exclusion of any other sexual act. He had sex with his wife, but only to please her. Dr. Tobin diagnosed him with severe pedophilia.

3. As a young boy, Shawn was treated harshly by his father and neglected by his mother. He longed for his father's approval and felt outraged at having been made to feel so worthless. He suppressed his feelings of powerlessness. He may have been sexually abused. His volunteer work with young boys was, to him, a way of helping boys in need. He identified with the young boys and did not see them as different from himself, though he was many years older than they were.

4. Dr. Tobin admitted Shaun into an outpatient treatment program, which consisted of intensive individual and group therapy, as well as aversion therapy aimed at reducing and eventually eliminating his sexual responsiveness to children. He responded well to aversion therapy but was slower to come to terms with his problems in group and individual therapy. When he finally admitted that a neighbor had sexually abused him when he was 12, he started to gain some insight into his own behavior as repetitive of what he had experienced. He continued in therapy for years and then left the state to start a new life.

REVIEW AT A GLANCE

1. causes harm to others
2. persistent or recurrent distress; impairment in important areas of functioning
3. Paraphilias
4. six
5. nonhuman objects
6. children or other nonconsenting persons
7. the suffering or humiliation by self or partner
8. Pedophilia
9. sixteen
10. sexually immature children
11. exhibitionism
12. intense sexual urges; arousing fantasies
13. genital exposure to strangers
14. fetishism
15. object
16. sexual gratification
17. frotteur
18. rubbing against
19. fondling
20. Sexual masochism
21. painful stimulation applied to one's own body
22. Sexual sadism
23. harm another person
24. Transvestic fetishism
25. wear a woman's clothing; cross-dressing
26. Voyeurism
27. observing the nudity or sexual activity of others
28. adolescence
29. psychological factors
30. learning events
31. conditioned response
32. medication
33. psychotherapy
34. group; family
35. Gender identity disorder
36. assigned sex; gender identity
37. hormones
38. fetal development
39. a parent's preference for a child of the other gender
40. early attachment experiences
41. unintentional reinforcement of cross-gender behavior by parents
42. sex reassignment surgery
43. Sexual dysfunctions
44. responsiveness
45. reactions
46. hypoactive sexual desire disorder
47. Sexual aversion disorder
48. female sexual arousal disorder
49. Male erectile disorder
50. Female orgasmic disorder
51. male orgasmic disorder

52. premature ejaculation
53. Sexual pain disorders
54. dyspareunia
55. vaginismus
56. Dyspareunia
57. pain
58. Vaginismus
59. recurrent; persistent
60. physical
61. psychological
62. medication
63. behavioral
64. cognitive-behavioral
65. couples

MULTIPLE CHOICE

1. (a) is correct. (b), (c), and (d) would decrease the likelihood of sexual offending.
2. (b) is correct. There is no evidence for (a), (c), and (d).
3. (c) is correct. (a) involves looking at others; (b) the infliction of pain; and (d) objects or particular body parts.
4. (d) is correct. (a) involves preferring sex with children; (b) is forced sexual intercourse; (c) is a general term, not a diagnosis itself.
5. (a) is correct. (b) would be counterindicated; (c) and (d) are not used to treat this disorder.
6. (a) is correct. (b), (c), and (d) do not involve tying up a sexual partner.
7. (b) is correct. (a) involves dressing in women's clothing; (c) the inability to experience orgasm; and (d) sexual acts performed on one's self.
8. (a) is correct. (b), (c), and (d) are not necessarily related to postsurgical adjustment.
9. (a) is correct. (b) involves the extent to which one's behavior matches one's assigned sex; (c) the gender-based behavior itself; and (d) involves dressing and living as the opposite of your assigned sex.
10. (c) is correct. (a) involves sexual satisfaction through abnormal means; (b) does not specifically describe low interest level; and (d) is the inability to achieve orgasm.
11. (a) is correct. (b), (c) and (d) are all more true of murderers who have mood disorders
12. (d) is correct. (a) and (b) are psychological, not physical, states; and (c) describes vaginismus.
13. (c) is correct. (a) involves legal issues; (b) and (d) involve cultural and social standards.
14. (c) is correct. (a), (b), and (d) are not known to be associated with exhibitionism.
15. (a) is correct. (b), (c), and (d) describe other sexual disorders.
16. (b) is correct. (a) involves reconditioning by pairing sexual response with pain or discomfort; (c) is a cognitive method; and (d) is a form of couple's therapy.
17. (d) is correct. (a), (b), and (c) are not directly associated with abnormal sexual behaviors.
18. (a) is correct. There is no clear evidence in support of (b), (c), and (d).
19. (c) is correct. (a) involves male dysfunction; (b) and (d) have to do with level of desire.
20. (d) is correct. (a), (b), and (c) are not contributors to this therapeutic approach.
21. (d) is correct. (a), (b), and (c) are not required for paraphilias.
22. (a) is correct. (b), (c), and (d) do not fit the description of the person preferring children.
23. (b) is correct. (a) involves utilizing pain for the purposes of pleasure; (c) involves dressing as the other sex; and (d) involves dressing as the other sex.
24. (d) is correct. (a), (b), and (c) do not fit the described behavior, trying to enhance normal sexual performance.
25. (d) is correct. (a) involves sex with children; (b) looking at others in the sex act; and (c) sexual arousal from dressing as the opposite sex.
26. (d) is correct. (a) and (b) have to do with sexual desire; (c) is not a disorder.
27. (a) is correct. (b) and (c) involve problems in arousal and performance; (d) is a dislike for sex.
28. (c) is correct. (a) and (b) are not indicated by a flaccid penis; and (d) involves orgasm, not penile erection.
29. (d) is correct. (a) and (b) involve manipulating and prolonging sexual performance; (c) is a behavioral method used to treat some sexual disorders.
30. (d) is correct. (a), (b), and (c) do not match the described behaviors.

CHAPTER 8
MOOD DISORDERS

CHAPTER AT A GLANCE

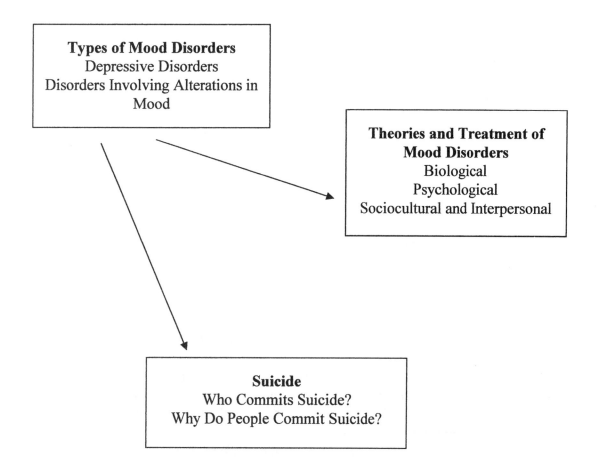

Types of Mood Disorders
Depressive Disorders
Disorders Involving Alterations in Mood

Theories and Treatment of Mood Disorders
Biological
Psychological
Sociocultural and Interpersonal

Suicide
Who Commits Suicide?
Why Do People Commit Suicide?

Learning Objectives

1.0   General Characteristics of Mood Disorders
     1.1   Define the nature of an episode as used to diagnose a mood disorder.
     1.2   Explain the severity of the episode with a specifier, such as, mild, moderate, or severe.

One Question

2.0   Depressive Disorders
     2.1   Indicate the diagnostic characteristics of a major depressive episode, types of depression, epidemiology, and course of major depressive disorder.
     2.2   Enumerate the criteria used to diagnose dysthymic disorder.

3.0   Disorders Involving Alternations in Moods
     3.1   Describe the symptoms of a manic episode, the types of bipolar disorder, epidemiology, and course of bipolar disorder.
     3.2   Indicate the diagnostic criteria for cyclothymic disorder.

4.0   Theories and Treatments of Mood Disorders
     4.1   Explain the biological perspective, including approaches to theory and treatment that focus on genetics and biochemical abnormalities.
     4.2   Evaluate the psychodynamic perspective and its application to understanding and treating mood disorders.
     4.3   Describe the behavioral perspective and how it is used to treat and understand mood disorders.
     4.4   Outline the cognitive-behavioral perspective of the nature and treatment of mood disorders.
     4.5   Clarify the nature of the sociocultural and interpersonal perspective of mood disorders and indicate how they are used in treatment.

5.0   Suicide
     5.1   Describe the characteristics of people who commit suicide.
     5.2   Compare and contrast the biological, psychological, and sociocultural perspectives of why people commit suicide ~~and outline the nature of assessment and treatment of suicidality~~.
     5.3   Outline the nature of the assessment and treatment of suicidality.

6.0   Mood Disorders: The Biopsychosocial Perspective
     6.1   Contrast and integrate the current approaches to mood disorders.

7.0   Chapter Box
     7.1   Discuss the case of Kay Redfield Jamison.

Identify the Theory

Put the letter corresponding to the theoretical perspective in the blank next to each proposed cause of depression:

P = Psychodynamic   **C** = Cognitive-behavioral
B = Behavioral   **I** = Interpersonal

Perspective	Cause of depression

1. _____ Distorted attitudes and perceptions of experiences.
2. _____ Criticism and rejection by others.
3. _____ Feelings of guilt and abandonment.
4. _____ Negative view of self, world, and future.
5. _____ Lack of intimate relationships
6. _____ Attributions of helplessness.
7. _____ Loss of loved object.
8. _____ Lack of positive reinforcement.
9. _____ Perceived loss, which diminishes self-esteem.
10. _____ Disruption of customary routines or scripts.

Matching

Put the letter from the right-hand column corresponding to the correct match in the blank next to each item in the left-hand column.

1. ___ Wonder drug of the 1990s.
2. ___ Lethargic and listless behavior.
3. ___ Medication most effective in treating bipolar disorder.
4. ___ Relatives with identical genetic makeup.
5. ___ Taking excessive responsibility for failures.
6. ___ Symptom of major depressive disorder.
7. ___ Treatment of depression that involves working through conflicts related to particular life concerns.
8. ___ Measurement of cortisol levels.
9. ___ Treatment of depression that involves changing dysfunctional thoughts.
10. ___ Response to ECT.
11. ___ Chronic and less intense form of depression.
12. ___ Explanations people have for the things that happen to them.
13. ___ Period of elevated and expansive mood.
14. ___ Chronic vacillation between states of euphoria and dysphoria.
15. ___ Variant of depression that has no external causes.

a. endogenous
b. attributions
c. cognitive restructuring
d. lithium
e. psychomotor retardation
f. manic episode
g. dysthymic disorder
h. monozygotic twins
i. DST
j. short-term dynamic psychotherapy
k. clonic phase
l. example of cognitive distortion
m. Prozac
n. dysphoria
o. cyclothymic disorder

Short Answer

1. What are five factors that predispose a person to recurrent depression?

   _____   _____
   _____   _____
   _____

2. From the point of view of the person experiencing a manic episode, what are two appealing and two disturbing features of such an experience?

Appealing features	Disturbing features

3. What are three reasons for the Amish being considered especially suitable to study for research on bipolar disorder?

   _____
   _____

4. What three lines of specific evidence are used to support genetic theories of mood disorders?

   _____
   _____
   _____

5. Describe the evidence indicating an interaction of genetic and environmental contributions to mood disorders, as indicated by research on adult female twins:

   _____
   _____
   _____

6. What two facts challenge the monoamine deficit hypothesis of depression?

   _____
   _____

7. People with major depressive disorder show what altered biological rhythms?

   _____
   _____
   _____
   _____

8. List two experimental methods for treating depression that involve altering biological rhythms, and explain the proposed method of action for each:

Treatment	Proposed method of action

9. Fill in the information in the following chart with the proposed mechanism of action, disorder for which it is applied, and problems involved in the use of each somatic treatment listed:

Treatment	Mechanism of action	Disorder	Problems
Tricyclic antidepressants			
MAOIs			
Prozac			
Lithium			
Electroconvulsive therapy			

10. Describe the following theories of suicide and the theorist who proposed the theory or the basis of support for the theory:

Theory	Description	Theorist or basis of support for theory
Anomie		
Communication		
Hopelessness		
Genetic		
Neurotransmitter		

Letterbox Puzzle

Find the words that fit the definitions below each of the puzzles. The words may be formed by choosing one block from each column. You may cross out squares as you solve, because each box is used only once.

DE	OS	ST	O	N	VE
E	P	I	S	MI	DE
S	E	AN	S	OL	UM
D	P	RE	HY	RT	C
P	Y	AS	PA	SI	IC
M	EL	T	CH	O	AL

Clues:

X   Period in which specific intense symptoms are present.

X   Type of depression involving loss of interest in activities, symptoms in the morning, significant disturbance of appetite and extreme feelings of guilt.

X   In major _____ disorder, the individual feels extreme dysphoria, has physical symptoms, experiences low self-esteem, and may be suicidal.

X   Depressive disorder involving chronic sadness without a period of intense symptoms.

X   Pattern of depression in which symptoms are worst during the fall or winter.

X   Specifier used to indicate depression in a woman that follows the birth of a child.

E	CL	P	Z	L	L
C	U	R	O	A	A
C	OG	PH	TH	RI	IC
P	O	O	TI	YM	VE
B	I	O	O	SO	C
CY	R	NI	T	I	AR

Clues:

X   Disorder involving intense alternations in mood involving manic and/or depressive episodes.

X   Hormone involved in mobilizing the body' resources in times of stress.

X   Medication used to treat depression by altering the serotonin system; considered the "wonder drug" of the 1990s.

X   According to one theory, people who are depressed experience a _____ triad of negative feelings about the self, the world, and the future.

X   Feelings of intense elation or positive mood.

X   Disorder involving chronic alternations in mood from mild depression to hypomania.

Focusing on Research

Answer the following questions from "Research Focus: Interpersonal Therapy for Depression."

1. Summarize the common research question shared by the studies.

_____

_____

2. What are the most reasonable conclusions that can be drawn from the studies concerning the relative effectiveness of medication, cognitive-behavioral therapy, and interpersonal therapy to treat depression?

_____

_____

3. What specific questions remain about the conditions that facilitate effectiveness of interpersonal therapy and medication in treating depression?

_____

_____

From the Case Files of Dr. Sarah Tobin: Thinking About Janice's Case

Answer the following questions about the case of Janice Butterfield.

1. Outline the history of Janice's illness and treatment as reported to Dr. Tobin by Dr. Hampden.

_____

_____

_____

2. Describe Dr. Tobin's assessment of Janice's case and her diagnosis.

_____

_____

_____

3. What was Dr. Tobin's formulation of Janice's case?

_____

_____

_____

4. Describe the course and outcome of Janice's treatment.

_____

_____

_____

Review at a Glance

Test your knowledge by completing the blank spaces with terms from the chapter. If you need a hint, consult the chapter summary.

A mood disorder involves a disturbance in a person's (1) _____ or (2) _____. People can experience this disturbance in the form of (3) _____, (4) _____, or a (5) _____. An (6) _____ is a time-limited period during which specific intense symptoms of a disorder are evident. (7)_____ involves acute but time-limited episodes of depressive symptoms, such as feelings of (8) _____, a loss of interest in (9) _____, (10) _____ symptoms, and disturbances in (11) _____ and _____ behavior. Individuals with major depressive disorder also have cognitive symptoms, such as a negative (12) _____, feelings of (13) _____, an inability to (14) _____, and (15)_____. Depressive episodes are either (16) _____ or (17) _____. People with (18) _____ disorder have, for at least (19) _____ years, depressive symptoms such as low (20) _____, low (21) _____, poor (22) _____, (23) _____ difficulty, feelings of (24) _____, and disturbances of (25) _____ and _____.

(26)_____ disorder involves intense experiences of elation or euphoria called a (27) _____, characterized by heightened levels of (28) _____, (29) _____, and (30) _____. A mixed episode consists of symptoms of both a (31) _____ episode and a (32) _____ episode, which alternate rapidly. (33)_____ disorder involves a vacillation between (34)_____ and (35)_____ episodes. (36)_____ disorder involves one or more manic episodes sometimes (but not always) with one or more (37)_____ episodes. In bipolar II disorder, the individual has had (38) _____ major depressive episodes and at least (39) _____ hypomanic episode.

Biological theories explaining mood disorders focus on (40) _____ and (41) _____ functioning. Psychological theories emphasize the (42) _____, (43) _____ and (44) _____, aspects of mood disturbance. From the behavioral viewpoint, depression is the result of a reduction in (45) _____, deficient (46) _____, or (47) _____. According to the cognitive perspective, depressed people react to stressful experiences with a way of thinking called the (48) _____, a negative view of (49) _____, (50) _____, and (51) _____. (52)_____ are errors in the way people draw conclusions from their experiences, applying illogical rules such as (53)

_____ or (54) _____ . (55)_____ theory emphasizes disturbed social functioning.

Biological treatments for depression include mostly (56) _____ and, for extreme cases, (57) _____ . (58)_____ is the most widely used medication for bipolar disorder. Psychological interventions involve the (59)_____ and (60) _____methods. Sociocultural and interpersonal interventions focus on treatment within the context of an (61) _____ system, such as an (62) _____ relationship.

Many suicidal people have a (63) _____disorder, and some suffer from other serious (64) _____ disorders. Most interventions incorporate (65) _____ and (66) _____ methods.

Multiple Choice

1. Suicide hot lines may not be effective because
   a. they are often poorly funded and staffed.
   b. callers do not divulge their identity.
   c. they are staffed by under trained people.
   d. people do not call when at highest risk.

2. A diagnosis of bipolar disorder requires
   a. the experience of a depressive episode.
   b. the experience of a manic episode.
   c. a family history of mood disorder.
   d. normal premorbid personality.

3. The suicide rate is highest among white males aged
   a. 15 to 24.
   b. 30 to 40.
   c. 50 to 65.
   d. 85 or older.

4. Which of the following factors indicates that a suicide case should be viewed as high-risk?
   a. an elaborate suicide plan
   b. low suicidal lethality
   c. low suicidal intention
   d. parasuicidal intent

5. People with cyclothymic disorder experience chronic
   a. episodes of depression.
   b. episodes of mania.
   c. alterations from dysphoria to hypomania.
   d. unrelenting hypomania.

6. Which statement is true regarding the role of genetics in mood disorders?
   a. In families in which one parent has a mood disorder, between 60 percent and 70 percent of offspring are likely to develop a mood disorder.
   b. Among dizygotic twins, the concordance rate is between 45 percent and 50 percent.
   c. Among monozygotic twins, the concordance rate is between 65 percent and 70 percent.
   d. In families in which both parents have mood disorders, between 90 percent and 95 percent of their offspring are likely to develop a mood disorder.

7. A psychiatrist has determined that a client has bipolar disorder. Of the following, which kind of medication is most likely to be prescribed?
   a. lithium carbonate
   b. tricyclics
   c. MAOIs
   d. anticonvulsants

8. The popularity of fluoxetine (Prozac) as a treatment of depression is due to the fact that Prozac is
   a. economical.
   b. impressively effective with few side effects.
   c. so aggressively marketed.
   d. targeted to a wide range of neurotransmitters.

9. According to Seligman's learned helplessness theory, depressed people
   a. view themselves as incapable of having an effect on their environment.
   b. take comfort in the attention they receive from others.
   c. tend to exaggerate their symptoms in order to get out of undesirable responsibilities.
   d. have negative views of self, world, and future.

10. Dr. Charney is a cognitive-behavioral therapist. She is least likely to use which approach?
    a. cognitive restructuring
    b. didactic work
    c. graded task assignments
    d. electroconvulsive therapy

11. Catecholamine is to _____ as indolamine is to _____
    a. serotonin; norepinephrine.
    b. GABA; serotonin.
    c. norepinephrine; serotonin.
    d. dopamine; norepinephrine.

12. In an important NIMH study comparing the relative effectiveness of medications and psychotherapy, Elkin and his colleagues concluded that people with
    a. severe depression benefited most from cognitive behavioral therapy alone
    b. mild depression benefited most from small doses of antidepressant medication.
    c. severe depression benefited from neither medication nor psychotherapy
    .d. mild depression benefited nearly equally from medication, cognitive-behavioral therapy, and interpersonal psychotherapy.

13. In the textbook case of Janice Butterfield, Dr. Tobin noted that Janice's WAIS-R scores reflected her serious depression. Which of the following would have led Dr. Tobin to draw this conclusion?
    a. Lethargy caused Janice to receive a Performance IQ substantially below her Verbal IQ.
    b. Janice's vocabulary definitions were not particularly creative, thus causing her to receive a below average Verbal IQ.
    c. There was a negative correlation between Janice's IQ score and her MMPI-2 scores.

    d. Most of Janice's responses contained aspects of delusional thinking and bizarre associations.

14. Researchers find that there is a sizeable percentage of individuals suffering from depression who also have the symptoms of another psychological disorder. Which disorder is it?
    a. somatization disorder
    b. post-traumatic stress disorder
    c. anxiety disorder
    d. dissociative disorder

15. Researchers have proposed that the seasonal type of depression may be caused by alterations in biological rhythms due to seasonal variations in
    a. caloric intake.
    b. temperature.
    c. norepinephrine production.
    d. light.

16. Central to early psychodynamic explanations of depression is the notion of
    a. "loss" at an unconscious level.
    b. disordered thinking patterns.
    c. lack of positive reinforcement.
    d. regression to an egoless state.

17. Which of the following statements is true regarding the rate of depression in African Americans?
    a. It is generally higher than is found for Whites.
    b. The rates are highest for those in their twenties.
    c. The rates are highest for those in their forties.
    d. The rates of seasonal depression are higher than in Whites.

18. That depressed people may be hypersensitive to norepinephrine levels and that biochemical changes in their brains may have decreased their sensitivity to norepinephrine is related to the process of
    a. synergism.
    b. down-regulation.
    c. catecholamine deregulation.
    d. up-regulation.

19. An alternate somatic treatment for individuals suffering from severe depression who are not helped by medications is
    a. dexamethasone therapy.
    b. acetylcholamine therapy.
    c. electroconvulsive therapy.
    d. tricyclic antidepressant therapy.

20. The therapy derived from interpersonal theory follows a set of guidelines derived from
    a. case studies.
    b. empirical research.
    c. naturalistic observations.
    d. laboratory studies.

21. Terms such as mild, severe, in remission, and recurrent as they apply to mood disorders are referred to as
    a. designators.
    b. denoters.
    c. appliers.
    d. specifiers.

22. The theory that depression stems from a negative view of one's self, the world, and the future comes from which perspective?
    a. psychodynamic
    b. behavioral
    c. interpersonal
    d. cognitive-behavioral

23. Joe has a mood disorder in which he experiences alternating episodes of severe depression and mild bouts of mania. Which of the following diagnoses would best describe Joe's condition?
    a. bipolar I disorder
    b. bipolar II disorder
    c. manic depression
    d. cyclothymia

24. Major depression is to _____ as bipolar disorder is to _____.
    a. dysthymia; cyclothymia
    b. dysphoria; euphoria
    c. depression; mania
    d. dysphoria; hypothymia

25. The notion that low levels of norepinephrine cause depression and high levels cause mania is the basis of what is called the _____ hypothesis.
    a. catecholamine
    b. GABA
    c. adrenaline
    d. serotonin

26. Dr. Jaspers feels that Rhonda's manic episode is an unconscious defense she is using to guard against sinking into a state of gloom and despair. Based on this information Dr. Jaspers' orientation is most likely
    a. humanistic.
    b. behavioral.
    c. existential.
    d. psychodynamic.

27. The phenomenon that Seligman observed in dogs that were subjected to inescapable shock is referred to as
    a. cognitive distortion.
    b. volitional apathy.
    c. learned helplessness.
    d. conditioned hopelessness.

28. According to Aaron Beck's cognitive theory, errors that depressed people make in the way that they draw conclusions from their experiences are called
    a. attribution errors.
    b. delusions.
    c. cognitive distortions.
    d. cognitive misattributions.

29. Which theory connects the ideas of psychoanalytic theorists with the ideas of behavioral and cognitive theorists?
    a. interpersonal theory
    b. psychodynamic theory
    c. family/systems theory
    d. person-centered theory

30. Which type of antidepressant is prescribed less often than others due to its often fatal interactions with other drugs?
    a. SSRIs
    b. lithium carbonate
    c. MAOIs

d. tricyclic

Answers

IDENTIFYING THEORIES

1.	C	3.	P	5.	I	7.	P	9.	C
2.	I	4.	C	6.	C	8.	B	10.	B

MATCHING

1.	m	4.	h	7.	j	10.	k	13.	f
2.	e	5.	l	8.	i	11.	g	14.	o
3.	d	6.	n	9.	c	12.	b	15.	a

SHORT ANSWERS

1. History of past depressive episodes;
   recent stress;
   minimal social support;
   family history of depression;
   lifestyle, personality, and health behaviors.
2. Appealing features—Heightened energy; heightened creativity.
   Disturbing features—Irritability; lack of judgment.
3. They have restricted lineage.
   Careful genealogical records are kept.
   Their religion prohibits drug and alcohol use.
4. Higher concordance based on proximity of biological relationship, including clustering of disorders among families of probands.
   Family lineage studies that identify specific chromosomal abnormalities.
   Adoption studies showing higher concordance among biological than adoptive relatives.
5. Female twins with a genetic predisposition to depression who suffered a traumatic life event had a much higher rate of depression (15 percent) than female twins with no genetic predisposition to depression (6 percent). Female twins who did not experience a traumatic event had an equal rate of depression (about 1 percent) regardless of genetic predisposition.
6. Medications take at least 2 weeks to have effects.
   There is no evidence of a relationship between antihypertensive medication use (which reduces catecholamine activity) and depression.
7. Altered REM patterns, decreased time between falling asleep and REM sleep, earlier awakenings, seasonal variations in symptoms

8.

Treatment	Proposed method of action
Light therapy	Exposure to bright light reduces melatonin production by the pineal gland; this may relieve depression in some people.
Sleep deprivation	Altering a person's biological rhythm through sleep deprivation may alleviate depression and in some cases may increase the effects of antidepressant medication.

9.

Treatment	Mechanism of action	Disorder	Problems
Tricyclic antidepressants	Increase monoamine activity	Depression	Take at least 2 weeks to have effect. Not effective for all depressions.
MAOIs	Inhibit MAO	Depression	Take at least 2 weeks to have effect. Potentially dangerous side effects.
Prozac	Increase serotonin activity	Depression	Possible risks of increased impulsivity and suicide.
Lithium	Decreased catecholamine activity	Bipolar disorder	Potentially dangerous side effects. From client's perspective, interferes with "high."
Electroconvulsive therapy	Not known	Depression	Short-term memory loss. Adverse connotations.

10.

Theory	Description	Theorist or basis of support for theory
Anomie	Feeling of alienation from society leads individual to experience suicidal wishes.	Emil Durkheim
Communication	Suicide is an attempt at interpersonal communication.	Edwin Shneidman
Hopelessness	Depression leads to unresolvable feelings of stress and hopelessness.	Aaron Beck
Genetic	Suicidal behavior has an inherited component.	Higher rates of concordance of suicidal behavior in identical compared with fraternal twins; adoption studies support the role of heredity.
Neuro-transmitter	Physiological differences exist between suicidal completers and controls.	Suicide victims found to have lower GABA levels in hypothalamus, lower serotonin levels.

LETTERBOX PUZZLE

Episode	Dysthymic	Bipolar	Cognitive
Melancholic	Seasonal	Cortisol	Euphoria
Depressive	Postpartum	Prozac	Cyclothymic

FOCUSING ON RESEARCH

1. The studies were designed to determine the relative effectiveness of interpersonal psychotherapy, cognitive behavioral psychotherapy, and medication for treating depression.
2. Generally, interpersonal psychotherapy and medication are equally effective for treating all kinds of depression, while cognitive-behavioral therapy is not as effective as medication.
3. We need to know specifically how interpersonal therapy and medication interact and how many sessions are

needed to achieve optimal therapeutic results.

FROM THE CASE FILES OF DR. SARAH TOBIN: THINKING ABOUT JANICE'S CASE

1. Janice had been seeing Dr. Hampden for 2 months. She appeared with complaints of exhaustion, sleep disturbance, lack of appetite, feelings of sadness and gloom, and interpersonal problems with her husband. Dr. Hampden prescribed Prozac, but Janice felt no better. The morning she was referred to Dr. Tobin, she attempted suicide by trying to asphyxiate herself in the car. Her husband found her and intervened.
2. Dr. Tobin conducted an interview, administered the MMPI-2, Rorschach, TAT, WAIS-III, and Beck Depression Inventory-II. Dr. Tobin diagnosed Janice with major depressive disorder.
3. Janice had unresolved conflicts over her mother's death, about which she felt relief and grief. Janice remained close to her mother long after her father's death when she was 14. Janice took care of her mother until she died, but she also felt resentment about doing so. When Janice's daughter became a toddler, the issues with her mother were reactivated. Being a mother thwarted her career goals and Janice felt resentment toward her husband.
4. Janice agreed to admit herself to the hospital where she remained for 3 weeks. She continued taking antidepressant medication and individual therapy with Dr. Tobin (who used cognitive-behavioral and psychodynamic techniques) as well as couples' therapy with one of Dr. Tobin's colleagues. Janice gained insight into the sources of her depression (which were biological and cognitive in origin), learned new ways of thinking about herself and her relationships, and improved communication with her husband. Janice's husband learned to relate differently to her and to better understand the impact of his behavior on Janice and their family.

REVIEW AT A GLANCE

1. emotional state
2. mood
3. extreme depression
4. excessive elation
5. combination of depression and elation
6. episode
7. Major depressive disorder
8. extreme dejection
9. previously pleasurable aspects of life
10. bodily
11. eating; sleeping
12. self-view
13. guilt
14. concentrate
15. indecisiveness
16. melancholic
17. seasonal
18. dysthymic
19. two
20. energy
21. self-esteem
22. concentration
23. decision-making
24. hopelessness
25. appetite; sleep
26. Bipolar
27. manic episode
28. thinking
29. behavior
30. emotionality
31. manic
32. major depressive
33. Cyclothymic
34. dysphoria
35. hypomanic
36. Bipolar I
37. major depressive
38. one or more
39. one
40. neurotransmitter
41. hormonal
42. behavioral
43. cognitive
44. Interpersonal
45. positive reinforcements
46. social skills
47. stressful life experiences
48. cognitive triad
49. the self
50. the world
51. the future
52. Cognitive distortions
53. arbitrary inferences
54. overgeneralizing
55. Interpersonal
56. antidepressant medication
57. electroconvulsive therapy
58. Lithium carbonate
59. behavioral
60. cognitive
61. interpersonal
62. intimate
63. mood
64. psychological
65. support
66. directive

MULTIPLE CHOICE

1. (d) is correct. While (b) may be true, that does not decrease their effectiveness; (a) and (c) are not true.
2. (b) is correct. (a), (c), and (d) are not required.
3. (d) is correct. (a) is the next highest rate, followed by (b) and (c).

4. (a) is correct. (b) and (c) mitigate against risk; (d) is also significant, but not as much as (a).
5. (c) is correct. (a), (b), and (d) are incorrect because cyclothymia involves alterations in mood.
6. (c) is correct. There is no empirical evidence to support (a), (b), and (d).
7. (a) is correct. (b) and (c) are used for depression; (d) may sometimes be used with lithium to treat bipolar.
8. (b) is correct. (a) and (d) are incorrect; (c) is true but that is not why it is a popular treatment.
9. (a) is correct. (b), (c), and (d) do not describe the disorder.
10. (d) is correct. (a), (b), and (c) are cognitive-behavioral approaches
11. (c) is correct. (a), (b), and (d) do not match the given analogy.
12. (d) is correct. The evidence did not support (a), (b), and (c).
13. (a) is correct. The assessment did not indicate (b), (c), or (d).
14. (c) is correct. (a), (b), (d) are not experienced by a sizeable number of people with depression.
15. (d) is correct. (a), (b), and (c) are not supported by evidence.
16. (a) is correct. (b) is a cognitive perspective; (c) a behavioral perspective; (d) is not representative of the psychodynamic or other perspectives.
17. (b) is correct. There is no evidence to support (a), (c), and (d).
18. (b) is correct. (a), (c), and (d) do not fit the described process.
19. (c) is correct. (a) and (d) are medications; (b) is not a medication regimen for depression.
20. (b) is correct. (a), (c), and (d) are not research methods used to test interpersonal therapy.
21. (d) is correct. (a), (b), and (c) do not describe the indicated terms.
22. (d) is correct. (a) believes that the roots of depression is in conflicting psychological processes stemming from childhood; (b) believes that depression is learned; and (c) is an integrative theory combining cognitive, behavioral, and psychodynamic perspectives.
23. (b) is correct. Hypomania is indicative of Bipolar II (a), (c), and (d) do not necessarily include the described phases.
24. (a) is correct. (b), (c), and (d) do not fit the described analogy.
25. (a) is correct. (b), (c), and (d) are neurotransmitters, but not implicated in the catecholamine hypothesis.
26. (d) is correct. (a), (b), and (c) would not have this explanation for depression.
27. (c) is correct. (a) is a term used in the cognitive perspective; (b) and (d) are not terms describing a psychological process.
28. (c) is correct. (a) involves who and what people blame or credit for events in their lives; (b) is an irrational thought; (d) is not a term used to describe a psychological process.
29. (a) is correct. (b), (c), and (d) do not integrative theories.
30. (c) is correct. (a) is an antidepressant, but SSRIs have the least side effects of the antidepressants; (b) is prescribed for bipolar; (d) is not commonly used today because of other side effects and lethality in overdose.

CHAPTER 9
SCHIZOPHRENIA
AND RELATED DISORDERS

CHAPTER AT A GLANCE

Schizophrenia and Related Disorders

Characteristics of Schizophrenia
Phases
Symptoms
Types
Dimensions
Courses
Gender, Age, and Cultural Features

Theories and Treatment
Biological
Psychological
Sociocultural

Other Psychotic Disorders
Brief Psychotic Disorder
Schizophreniform Disorder
Schizoaffective Disorder
Delusional Disorder
Shared Psychotic Disorder

14. ___ Period following the active phase of schizophrenia in which there are continuing signs of disturbance.
15. ___ Measure of the degree to which family members criticize, express hostility, and become overconcerned about a family member with schizophrenia.

Answer Game

This puzzle is like the popular television game show in which contestants provide the question for answers within certain categories. To solve this puzzle, write in the question within each category that corresponds to each of the answers. The answers are arranged in approximately increasing order of difficulty so that a 100-point question is less difficult than a 400-point question. Try playing this game with a friend and see who receives the higher score.

Points	Theory	Treatment	Famous person(s)	Research Design
100	A: An explanation of schizophrenia that focuses on altered neurotransmitter functioning. Q:	A: A somatic form of treatment that causes seizures. Q:	A: French physician who first identified schizophrenia as a disease. Q:	A: Design used to determine whether people with identical genetic endowment have the same risk for disorders. Q:
200	A: Explanation of schizophrenia that focuses on disturbed modes of communication within the home. Q:	A: Therapeutic environment in which staff and other clients work as a community. Q:	A: Quadruplets in NIMH study of genetic contributions to schizophrenia. Q:	A: Design in which people are studied who are born of biological parents with a disorder but raised by non-disordered parents. Q:
300	A: Behavioral explanation that schizophrenia results when an individual is designated as having the disorder and then acts accordingly. Q:	A: Behavioral intervention in which clients learn to interact appropriately with others. Q:	A: Introduced the idea of a vulnerability or diathesis model of schizophrenia. Q:	A: Design in which people are studied who are born of non-disordered parents but raised by disordered parents. Q:
400	A: Model of schizophrenia that proposes an interaction of genetic vulnerability and environmental stress. Q:	A: Medications that have antipsychotic properties. Q:	A: American psychiatrist who was one of the founders of the Danish adoption studies. Q:	A: Design in which people born of disordered parents are followed over their lives or assessed on certain key diagnostic tests. Q:

Short Answers

1. List Bleuler's "4 A's" and relate them to the current terms or concepts that are used to describe the same phenomena:

4 A's	Current diagnostic term or concept

2. Place a number next to the following ideas regarding the nature of schizophrenia indicating their historical order:

____ Restriction of criteria for diagnosing schizophrenia to a few critical symptoms that are clearly psychotic.

____ Distinction between Type I and Type II schizophrenia based on the nature of symptoms and other critical signs.

____ Schizophrenia defined as dementia praecox and regarded as due to premature brain degeneration.

____ Suggestion made that certain "first-rank" symptoms must be present for diagnosis of schizophrenia to be made.

____ Disorder labeled "schizophrenia" indicating that it was due to a split of psychic functions.

____ Schizophrenia identified as due to a form of disease.

3. List and define the symptoms of schizophrenia, and summarize the potential impact on the individual of each:

Symptom	Potential impact

4. Three ways of classifying schizophrenia were described in the text. Describe the rationale and arguments against each basis of classification.

Basis of classification	Rationale in support of this classification	Arguments against this classification
Paranoid/catatonic/ disorganized/residual/ undifferentiated		
Positive-negative dimension		
Process-reactive dimension		

5. For each of the three disorders listed below, summarize the current explanations of the disorder and methods of treatment as described in the text:

Disorder	Current explanations	Treatment
Schizophreniform disorder		
Schizoaffective disorder		
Shared psychotic disorder		

6. For these biological explanations of schizophrenia, describe the proposed mechanism of action, original evidence to support the explanation, criticisms about it, and current understanding:

Explanation	Dopamine hypothesis	Chromosomal abnormality
Mechanism of action		
Supportive evidence		
Criticisms		
Current understanding		

7. For each of the following methods of studying genetic vs. environmental influences on schizophrenia, describe what it is intended to show and what the limitations of the method are:

Method	Purpose	Limitations
Family concordance		
Twin studies		
Discordant twin-offspring study		
Adoption study		
Cross-fostering study		

8. Place an "X" next to the term that does not belong with the others:

a. Transactional
   Double-bind
   Labeling
   Expressed emotion

b. Cross-fostering
   Increased ventricle size
   Abnormal PET scans
   Cortical atrophy

c. Token economy
   Neuroleptics
   Social skills
   Milieu therapy

d. Sustained attention
   Smooth-pursuit eye movements
   Event-related potential
   Schizophrenia spectrum

e. High-risk
   Diathesis-stress
   Dopamine hypothesis
   Vulnerability

9. Answer the following questions regarding the case of the Genain quadruplets:

a. At what point in their lives did each of the sisters develop symptoms of schizophrenia?

_____

_____

b. What makes the study of the Genains so valuable in terms of understanding the causes of schizophrenia?

_____

_____

_____

c. What was the hypothesized role of Mrs. Genain in contributing to the illness of her daughters, and why is it necessary to interpret her role with caution?

_____

_____

_____

d. How did the 1981 follow-up status of the four quadruplets compare with their status at the earlier testing?

_____

_____

_____

e. What are the implications of the results from the Genain study for the study of genetic and environmental contributions to schizophrenia?

_____

_____

_____

Focusing on Research

Answer the following questions from "Research Focus: Can Delusions Be Changed?"

1. What is the basis for the belief that people with schizophrenia can change the nature of their delusions?

_____

_____

_____

2. Name and describe the techniques that cognitive therapists are using to help people modify their delusions.

_____

_____

_____

From the Case Files of Dr. Sarah Tobin: Thinking About David's Case

Answer the following questions about the case of David Marshall.

1. Describe David as Dr. Tobin observed him in the emergency room.

_____

_____

2. Discuss Dr. Tobin's assessment and diagnosis of David.

_____

_____

3. Describe Dr. Tobin's formulation of David's case.

_____
_____

4. Discuss the nature of course of David's treatment.

_____
_____

How Are We Different?

Answer the following questions from the text box, "How People Differ: Schizophrenia and Social Class."

1. Compare the social causation and downward social drift hypothesis of schizophrenia.

_____
_____

2. How does the diathesis-stress model of mental illness contribute to the debate of the relationship between schizophrenia and social class?

_____
_____

3. What do we still need to know that might help explain the fact that these hypotheses may clarify the incidence of schizophrenia within a society, but not between societies?

_____
_____

Review at a Glance

Test your knowledge by completing the blank spaces with terms from the chapter. If you need a hint, consult the chapter summary.

Schizophrenia involves disturbances in (1)_____, (2)_____, (3)_____, (4)_____, (5)_____, (6)_____, and (7)_____ lasting at least (8)_____ months. Symptoms apparent during the active phase are (9) _____, (10) _____, (11) _____, (12) _____, and (13) _____. The active phase is often preceded by a (14) _____ phase and followed by a (15) _____ phase. The prodromal phase is characterized by maladaptive behaviors such as (16) _____, inability to (17) _____, (18) _____, (19) _____, (20) _____, (21) _____ and _____, (22) _____, odd (23) _____, and decreased (24) _____ and _____. The (25) _____ phase involves continuing indications of disturbance similar to the behaviors of the prodromal phase.

There are several types of schizophrenia. (26)_____ type is characterized by bizarre motor behaviors, while disorganized types consists of symptoms including disorganized

(27)_____, disturbed (28) _____, and (29)_____ or (30)_____ affect. People with the paranoid type are preoccupied with one or more bizarre (31) _____ or have (32) _____ related to a theme of being persecuted or harassed. The diagnosis of (33) _____ type is used when a person does not meet the criteria for paranoid, catatonic, or disorganized type. (34)_____ type applies to people who have been diagnosed with schizophrenia and show lingering signs of the disorder without psychotic symptoms.

Schizophrenia is also characterized along two dimensions, distinguished by symptoms, for instance, (35) _____ (known as Type I) and (36) _____ symptoms, such as lack of motivation (known as Type II). The (37) _____ dimension differentiates a disorder that appears gradually over time from that provoked by a precipitant.

Disorders like those of schizophrenia include (38)_____, (39)_____, (40)_____, (41)_____, and (42)_____. Presumably, people who have schizophrenia have a (43) _____ determined (44) _____ to developing schizophrenia that develops when certain (45) _____ conditions are in place. Biological researchers have focused on abnormalities of brain (46) _____ and _____, (47) _____ predispositions, biological (48) _____, and (49) _____ stressors. Current comprehensive models of care include (50) _____ treatments, psychological interventions primarily in the form of (51) _____ techniques, and sociocultural interventions that focus on (52) _____ therapy and (53) _____ involvement.

Multiple Choice

1. David Marshall's parents described to Dr. Tobin David's gradual deterioration during late adolescence, suggesting that David was experiencing
    a. prodromal signs of schizophrenia.
    b. the residual phase of schizophrenia.
    c. schizoaffective disorder.
    d. a delusional disorder.

2. The "Four A's" which Bleuler described as the fundamental features of schizophrenia are
    a. anomie, association, ambivalence, and autism.
    b. antagonism, affect, association, and autism.
    c. association, affect, ambivalence, and autism.
    d. affiliation, association, affect, and autism.

3. Smaller frontal lobes and limbic system structures are thought to relate to
    a. the negative subtype of schizophrenia.
    b. the positive subtype of schizophrenia.
    c. the presence of schizoaffective disorder.
    d. the reduced production of dopamine.

4. Edgar believes that his heart is being eaten away by worms, a delusion that fits into the category called
    a. somatic.
    b. persecutory.
    c. insertion.
    d. nihilistic.

5. Which of the following is <u>not</u> a recognized symptom of schizophrenia?
    a. disturbed interpersonal relating ability
    b. disturbed sleep patterns
    c. disturbance in sense of self
    d. disturbance of affect

6. Which term is used for a research design that studies children whose biological parents did not have schizophrenia, but whose rearing parents did?
    a. index adoption
    b. schizophrenic spectrum
    c. multifactorial
    d. cross-fostering

7. The diathesis-stress model of vulnerability to schizophrenia proposes that
    a. some people have a predisposition that places them at risk for developing a disorder if exposed to certain stressful life experiences.
    b. trauma or stress may affect a person's interaction with offspring in such a way as to cause them to be vulnerable to developing a disorder.
    c. a disorder can only develop in individuals who have been exposed to stress.
    d. the closer the genetic relationship to a person with a disorder, the greater the likelihood of developing that disorder.

8. Soon after beginning a new and stressful job, Jason began to act in strange ways such as sending email messages to co-workers regarding life on other planets. After three months, Jason was given a medical leave and with treatment, returned to normal functioning. The most likely diagnosis for Jason would be
    a. brief psychotic disorder.
    b. schizophreniform disorder.
    c. reactive schizophrenia.
    d. schizoaffective disorder.

9. The symptoms of schizophrenia are associated mainly with the overactivity of neurons that respond to which neurotransmitter?
    a. norepinephrine
    b. GABA
    c. serotonin
    d. dopamine

10. Janet and Jeannine have a close but extremely paranoid relationship. Over the years they have come to fuel each other's delusional thinking. This condition is called
    a. shared psychotic disorder.
    b. delusional disorder, jealous type.
    c. shared schizophrenia.
    d. delusional disorder, grandiose type.

11. Emil Kraepelin believed that "dementia praecox" resulted from
    a. lengthy institutionalization.
    b. deterioration of the brain.
    c. disturbed parent-child relationships.
    d. impaired cognitive capacity.

12. Disorders involving the single psychotic symptom of false beliefs are called
    a. shared psychotic disorders.
    b. schizophreniform disorders.
    c. delusional disorders.
    d. factitious disorders.

13. *DSM-I* and *DSM-II*'s definitions of schizophrenia were
    a. very broad and resulted in overdiagnosis.
    b. too specific and narrow.
    c. stereotyped against minorities.
    d. not based on theory.

14. The case of the Genain quadruplets who developed schizophrenia provided evidence regarding the
    a. difference between Type 1 and Type 2 schizophrenia.
    b. role of dopamine in the development of schizophrenia.
    c. interaction of genetic and environmental factors in the development of schizophrenia.
    d. cross-fostering of schizophrenic traits among siblings.

15. Efforts by researchers to alter the nature and frequency of delusions in people with schizophrenia have shown that
    a. successful treatment required two to three years of intensive therapy.
    b. the greatest success resulted from reality testing exercises.
    c. although delusions decreased, subjects became more depressed and anxious.
    d. verbal challenges were most successful in promoting change.

16. According to the downward social drift hypothesis of schizophrenia:
    a. there is a decrease in the amount of brain processing of social input.
    b. people with schizophrenia develop the disorder because of low social class.
    c. after people develop schizophrenia, their social class declines.
    d. the friends of people with schizophrenia abandon them after they are diagnosed.

17. Which type of schizophrenia is characterized by incoherence, loose associations, inappropriate affect and haphazard behavior?
    a. paranoid type
    b. undifferentiated type
    c. catatonic type
    d. disorganized type

18. Researchers refer to the symptoms of schizophrenia that are exaggerations or distortions of normal thoughts, emotions, and behavior as:
    a. positive symptoms.
    b. negative symptoms.
    c. anhedonic symptoms.
    d. hebephrenic symptoms.

19. Which factor is NOT associated with favorable prognosis in schizophrenia?
    a. slow, gradual onset
    b. later age of onset
    c. being female
    d. good insight

20. The index of the degree that family members speak in ways that reflect criticism, hostile feelings, and emotional over-involvement or overconcern with regard to the individual with schizophrenia is referred to as:
    a. event related potential.
    b. expressed emotion.
    c. expressive threshold.
    d. affective index.

21. The Swiss psychiatrist who abandoned the term "dementia praecox" for the current label schizophrenia was
    a. Emil Kraepelin.
    b. Eugen Bleuler.
    c. Adolf Meyer.
    d. Benedict Morel.

22. For the past three months, Tom's speech has been gradually deteriorating and becoming incoherent, and he has been exhibiting purposeless and stereotyped behaviors. His symptoms at this point are not extremely active. In what phase of schizophrenia might Tom be at this point?
    a. residual phase
    b. active phase
    c. remission phase
    d. prodromal phase

23. Lori has a constant sensation that she has snakes crawling through her intestines. Lori is experiencing a(n)
    a. hallucination.
    b. delusion.
    c. apparition.
    d. chimera.

24. Even while talking about the death of her husband a decade ago, Carol giggles almost uncontrollably. Many people in the hospital characterize her as being silly. What type of schizophrenia might she have?
    a. undifferentiated schizophrenia
    b. disorganized schizophrenia
    c. catatonic schizophrenia
    d. paranoid schizophrenia

25. The type of schizophrenia involving a complex set of symptoms such as delusions, hallucinations, and incoherence, but in which no one symptom predominates is referred to as
    a. paranoid schizophrenia.
    b. undifferentiated schizophrenia.
    c. catatonic schizophrenia.
    d. disorganized schizophrenia.

26. Which term is used to refer to the gradual emergence of schizophrenia over time?
    a. process
    b. reactive
    c. acute
    d. chronic

27. Which of the following statements best characterizes the current thinking regarding recovery from schizophrenia?
    a. No one actually ever recovers from schizophrenia; the best to hope for is long-term symptom management.
    b. Total recovery in all cases of schizophrenia is possible with the proper medication.
    c. Recovery rates vary widely based on how narrowly the researcher defines recovery.
    d. Long-term hospitalization is necessary in most cases; even then the prognosis is uncertain.

28. Jennifer recently experienced a brief psychotic episode soon after her miscarriage. The symptoms lasted only about a month. Jennifer had experienced
    a. schizophreniform disorder.
    b. schizoid personality disorder.
    c. brief psychotic disorder.
    d. disorganized schizophrenia.

29. The fact that antipsychotic drugs reduce the frequency of the symptoms of schizophrenia provides evidence for the
    a. dopamine hypothesis.
    b. hemispheric dominance hypothesis.
    c. frontal lobe atrophy hypothesis.
    d. serotonin hypothesis.

30. A disturbance in which of the following is one of the biological markers for schizophrenia?
    a. smooth pursuit eye movements
    b. divided attention
    c. expressed emotion
    d. event related potential

Answers

IDENTIFYING DISORDERS

1. Schizophrenia
2. Brief psychotic disorder
3. Delusional disorder, jealous type
4. Schizophrenia, paranoid type
5. Delusional disorder, erotomanic type
6. Schizophrenia, undifferentiated type
7. Schizophrenia, catatonic type
8. Delusional disorder, persecutory type
9. Schizophrenia, disorganized type
10. Schizoaffective disorder
11. Schizophreniform disorder
12. Shared psychotic disorder

MATCHING

1. n
2. j
3. i
4. f
5. h
6. m
7. a
8. o
9. g
10. d
11. e
12. c
13. b
14. k
15. l

ANSWER GAME

Categories

Question Value	Theory	Treatment	Famous Person or People	Research Design
100	What is the dopamine hypothesis?	What is ECT?	Who is Benjamin Morel?	What is a twin study?
200	What is family systems?	What is milieu therapy?	Who are the Genain sisters?	What is an adoption study?
300	What is labeling?	What is social skills training?	Who is Paul Meehl?	What is cross-fostering?

400	What is diathesis-stress?	What are neuro-leptics?	Who is Seymour Kety?	What is a high-risk study?

SHORT ANSWER

1.

4 A's	Current diagnostic term or concept
Association	Incoherence
Affect	Disturbance of affect
Ambivalence	Disturbance of motivation
Autism	Disturbed interpersonal relating ability

2. 5, 6, 2, 4, 3, 1

3.

Symptom	Potential impact
Disturbance of thought content: Delusions	Misinterpret behavior of others; form erroneous conclusions from daily experiences.
Disturbance in perceptions: Hallucinations	Images may be frightening and painful and are disruptive in daily life. May include "commands" that result in harm to others.
Disturbance of thinking, language, and communication: Disorganized speech	Difficulties in social interactions.
Disturbed behavior	Behavior looks odd to other people.
Negative symptoms	Loss of spontaneity and enjoyment in daily life, including the ability to experience pleasure from activities.
Social and occupational dysfunction	Lack of interaction with others causes loss of social skills which leads to further isolation; inability to keep a job influences standard of living.

4.

Basis of classification	Rationale in support of this classification	Arguments against this classification
Paranoid/catatonic/ disorganized/residual/ undifferentiated	Captures qualitative differences based on symptoms.	Categories do not capture underlying dimensions of schizophrenia.
Positive-negative dimension	Reliable system for predicting long-term outcome.	Difficult to form clear-cut diagnosis and many clients have "mixed" symptoms.
Process-reactive dimension	Intended to provide a useful system for diagnosis and estimation of prognosis.	People with symptoms on reactive pole of dimension no longer regarded as having a diagnosis of schizophrenia.

5.

Disorder	Current explanations	Treatment
Schizophreniform disorder	Biological links to schizophrenia as indicated by large brain ventricles, similar PET scans, and higher incidence in biological relatives.	Antipsychotic medications, antianxiety medications, lithium, ECT, and psychotherapy.
Schizoaffective disorder	Schizophrenia-like symptoms in addition to severe mood disturbances. Debate over whether disorder is a variant of schizophrenia or affective disorder.	Lithium, antidepressant medications, antipsychotic medications, and psychotherapy.
Shared psychotic disorder	Relationship issues in which dominant person feels isolated and seeks ally in weaker person who has come to rely on the other. Submissive person comes to hold beliefs of the dominant person	Separation of the two individuals; therapy with submissive partner regarding vulnerability to domination.

6.

Explanation	Dopamine hypothesis	Chromosomal abnormality
Mechanism of action	Increased dopamine activity.	Defect on a given chromosome underlies dopamine abnormality.
Supportive evidence	Antipsychotic drugs block dopamine receptors. Drugs related to dopamine increase frequency of psychotic symptoms.	Genetic mapping studies involving attempts to identify a susceptibility gene for schizophrenia have indicated several possible loci.
Criticisms	No difference exists between people with schizophrenia and normal individuals in dopamine metabolism.	Original findings have not been reliably replicated by other investigators.
Current understanding	Dopamine hypothesis may apply to Type 1 schizophrenia but not Type 2.	Researchers are still hoping to discover chromosomal abnormalities related to schizophrenia.

7.

Method	Purpose	Limitations
Family concordance	Relationship between proximity of biological relationship and concordance for schizophrenia.	Families share not only genetics factors but also the same environments.
Twin studies	Identical twins share same genetic endowment; concordance rate for schizophrenia reveals direct estimate of genetic contribution.	Identical twins share the same environment as well as identical genetic makeup.
Discordant twin-offspring study	Determination of whether offspring of discordant twins have higher concordance for schizophrenia provides further information on genetic determination of the disorder.	Still remaining unclear is why in the original discordant pairs, one twin and not the other develops schizophrenia.
Adoption study	Rule out the influence of environmental factors in family concordance studies.	Adopting families may not be free of disorder and therefore not provide a "clean" environment.
Cross-fostering study	Evaluate the effect of environmental contributions to schizophrenia in the absence of genetic inheritance.	Very difficult to conduct due to small incidence of disordered adopting parents.

8.   a. Labeling   Family systems explanations of schizophrenia.
       b. Cross-fostering   Brain changes.
       c. Neuroleptics   Behavioral treatments for schizophrenia.
       d. Schizophrenia spectrum   Biological markers for schizophrenia.
       e. Dopamine hypothesis   Concepts related to the vulnerability model of schizophrenia.

9.   a. All showed signs of disorder by the time they were in their 20s as diagnosed by psychiatrists or NIMH experimenters.
     b. As identical quadruplets, they shared the same genetic makeup; it is unusual to find such a family. In addition, they were studied over the course of their adult lives.
     c. Mrs. Genain was hypothesized to have given conflicting and confusing messages to her daughters, and to pressure the more competent ones to conform to the characteristics of the sisters who had more severe disturbance. It is necessary to interpret Mrs. Genain's role with caution, because it would be a mistake to place too much importance on the effects of parenting style on the development of schizophrenia.
     d. The four sisters changed in order of degree of impairment with Hester and Iris originally showing more impairment than Nora and Myra; in the follow-up, Myra and Iris showed less impairment than the other two sisters.
     e. The fact that they all developed schizophrenia is convincing evidence for genetic contributions to the disorder; but the fact that their symptoms emerged in different ways over the years of adulthood, and that their relative degree of impairment shifted suggests an interaction of genetics with environmental factors.

FOCUSING ON RESEARCH

1. Researchers believe that delusions are attributions or judgments that people make in an effort to make sense of particular experiences or perceptions. Individuals with schizophrenia may develop delusions to bring order and understanding to unusual, frightening, or hallucinatory experiences.
2. Cognitive therapists use verbal challenge and reality testing. In verbal challenge, they examine the evidence supporting or contradicting the delusional beliefs and develop explanations that are more accurate and realistic. In reality testing, the therapist has clients carry out activities aimed at invalidating the delusion.

FROM THE CASE FILES OF DR. SARAH TOBIN: THINKING ABOUT DAVID'S CASE

1. David was yelling about wanting to see Zoroaster. He said he had been appointed to protect the world from evil forces, and that he was bearing a message of salvation.
2. David was experiencing hallucinations and delusions, so Dr. Tobin could on conduct a 30-minute mental status examination. All of his answers focused on his beliefs about Zoroaster and aliens, including his name and the date. He had loose associations and bizarre behaviors. He was impaired in most areas of everyday functioning. He was socially isolated and failed to take care of his personal hygiene. Dr. Tobin diagnosed him as having the undifferentiated type schizophrenia.
3. David's aunt probably was a schizophrenic. David had been withdrawn most of his life, unlike his outgoing brother (to whom his parents gave most of their attention). The message David got from his parents was that they were not as concerned with him as with his brother.
4. Dr. Tobin recommended that David remain in the hospital for 3 months and be treated with antipsychotic medication. His hospital course went well after he was stabilized on medication. Upon discharge from the hospital, he attended a day treatment program for 12 months. He then got a job at the library and did well, gaining a promotion that involved a lot of contact with the public. However, the stress of exposure to many people caused him to relapse. Within 2 weeks of starting his new position, he had a full-blown psychotic episode and went back to the hospital. After a short stay, he went back to the day treatment program for 6 months, and then agreed to move out of his parents' home into a group home for schizophrenics. He was able to go back to work. Dr. Tobin has seen him once a month for several years, and David has remained stable. However, David does not seem to be getting much of out psychotherapy.

HOW ARE WE DIFFERENT?

1. According to the social causation hypothesis, membership in lower socioeconomic classes may cause schizophrenia, because members of these classes experience highly stressful environmental factors that may be conducive to the development of schizophrenia. Individuals in lower socioeconomic classes experience numerous economic hardships, do not have access to high-quality education, health care, and employment, and may experience discrimination. The downward social drift hypothesis downplays the effects of socioeconomic stresses in the development of the disorder, but says that once people develop the disorder, their economic standing and social fortunes decline precipitously, in effect leading them into a lower socioeconomic class.

2. The social causation hypothesis is consistent with the "stress" component of the diathesis-stress model (that environmental stressors contribute to manifestation of a disorder). But the diathesis-stress model holds that there is a biological/genetic predisposition to schizophrenia, and that stressors trigger the onset of the disease.

3. We need to know more about societal values and beliefs about mental illness that lead to differing criteria for diagnosis.

REVIEW AT A GLANCE

1. thought
2. perception
3. affect
4. sense of self
5. motivation
6. behavior
7. interpersonal functioning
8. six
9. delusions
10. hallucinations
11. disorganized speech
12. disturbed behavior
13. negative symptoms
14. prodromal
15. residual
16. social withdrawal
17. work productively
18. eccentricity
19. poor grooming
20. inappropriate emotionality
21. peculiar thought and speech
22. unusual beliefs
23. perceptual experiences
24. energy/initiative
25. residual
26. catatonic
27. speech
28. behavior
29. flat
30. inappropriate
31. delusions
32. auditory hallucinations
33. undifferentiated
34. residual
35. positive
36. negative
37. process-reactive
38. brief psychotic disorder
39. schizophreniform disorder
40. schizoaffective disorder
41. delusional disorder
42. shared psychotic disorder
43. biologically
44. predisposition
45. environmental
46. structure; function
47. genetic
48. markers
49. biological
50. biological
51. behavioral
52. milieu
53. family

MULTIPLE CHOICE

1. (a) is correct. (b) refers to lingering symptoms after a period of active schizophrenia; (c) and (d) are not associated with gradual deterioration.
2. (c) is correct. (a) in incorrect, because anomie is not a feature; (b) because antagonism is not one; and (d) because affiliation is not a symptom.
3. (a) is correct. (b) is associated with increased dopamine levels, thus (d) is also incorrect; (c) is not associated with organic brain differences.
4. (a) is correct. (b) involves thoughts; (c) is not a form of delusion; and (d) involves feelings of nonexistence
5. (b) is correct. (a), (c), and (d) are recognized symptoms
6. (d) is correct. (a), (b), and (c) are not types of research design.
7. (a) is correct. (b) and (c) are inaccurate statements; (d) concerns concordance rates.
8. (b) is correct. Schizophreniform disorder involves disturbances lasting one to six months. (a) lasts between one day to one month, (c), and (d) are incorrect because they do not describe temporary conditions.
9. (d) is correct. Dopamine has been the most widely neurotransmitter in relation to schizophrenia. Studies of GABA (b), and serotonin (c) are still being done. There is no evidence of effects of norepinephrine (a) in schizophrenia.
10. (a) is correct. There is no evidence that they are grandiose or jealous delusions (b) and (d); there is not such

disorder as (c).

11. (b) is correct. (a), (c), and (d) are not related to Kraepelin's term or to his theory of schizophrenia.
12. (c) is correct. (a) involves more than one person; (b) has a range of symptoms; (d) is not a psychotic disorder.
13. (a) is correct. (b), (c), and (d) are inaccurate.
14. (c) is correct. (d) involves a research design not used in this case; (a) and (b) were not addressed in the research.
15. (d) is correct. (a), (b), and (c) have not been reported.
16. (c) is correct. (a) is not related to social factors; there is no evidence for (b); (d) may be true but it is not related to the downward drift hypothesis.
17. (d) is correct. (a), (b), and (c) are not characterized by these symptoms.
18. (a) is correct. (b) involves absence of speech and affect; (c) refers to a loss of enjoyment of life, more a factor in depression; and (d) is not a term in current use.
19. (a) is correct. (b), (c), and (d) are all associated with good prognosis, while (a) is not.
20. (b) is correct. (a) is a measure of cognitive activity; (c) and (d) are not terms used in the context of schizophrenia.
21. (b) is correct. (a) coined the term; (c) and (d) made other contributions.
22. (d) is correct. (a) occurs after an active phase; (b) is the presence of full-blown symptoms; and there is no such phase as (c).
23. (b) is correct. (a) involves perception; (c) and (d) are not terms used to describe schizophrenia symptoms.
24. (b) is correct. (a), (c), and (d) do not match the described symptoms.
25. (b) is correct. (a), (c), and (d) do not match the described symptoms.
26. (a) is correct. (b) involves onset as a reaction to some precipitant; (c) describes rapid onset of symptoms; and (d) is not used to describe the onset of schizophrenia.
27. (c) is correct. The course of the illness and response to treatment varies so that (a), (b), and (d) are not reasonable conclusions.
28. (c) is correct. (a) and (d) require longer expression of symptoms for a diagnosis; (b) is not a psychotic disorder.
29. (a) is correct. There is no serotonin hypothesis (d); (b) and (c) are unrelated to antipsychotic medication.
30. (a) is correct. (b) may be apparent in some clients, but it is a cognitive factor, not biological; (c) is a social factor stemming from family dynamics; and (d) is a measure of cognitive activity not necessarily related to schizophrenia.

CHAPTER **10**
PERSONALITY DISORDERS

CHAPTER AT A GLANCE

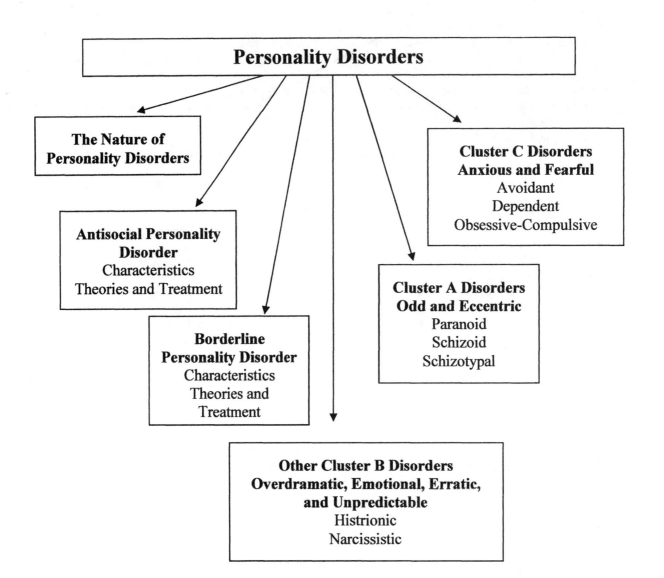

Personality Disorders

The Nature of Personality Disorders

Antisocial Personality Disorder
Characteristics
Theories and Treatment

Borderline Personality Disorder
Characteristics
Theories and Treatment

Other Cluster B Disorders
Overdramatic, Emotional, Erratic, and Unpredictable
Histrionic
Narcissistic

Cluster A Disorders
Odd and Eccentric
Paranoid
Schizoid
Schizotypal

Cluster C Disorders
Anxious and Fearful
Avoidant
Dependent
Obsessive-Compulsive

Learning Objectives

1.0   The Nature of Personality Disorders
      1.1   Describe the general features of a personality disorder as diagnosed in *DSM-IV-TR*.

2.0   Antisocial Personality Disorder
      2.1   Indicate the behaviors that are used to diagnose antisocial personality disorder.
      2.2   Contrast the biological, psychological, and sociocultural perspectives on understanding and treating antisocial personality disorder.

3.0   Borderline Personality Disorder
      3.1   Explain the characteristic features of borderline personality disorder.
      3.2   Compare the biological, psychological, and sociocultural theories and treatment of borderline personality disorder.

4.0   Histrionic Personality Disorder
      4.1   Describe the behaviors used to diagnose histrionic personality disorder.
      4.2   Contrast psychodynamic and cognitive-behavioral perspectives on this disorder and its treatment.

5.0   Narcissistic Personality Disorder
      5.1   Indicate the features used in the diagnosis of narcissistic personality disorder.
      5.2   Compare the approaches favored by psychodynamic and cognitive-behavioral approaches to understanding and treatment.

6.0   Paranoid Personality Disorder
      6.1   Explain the characteristic symptoms of paranoid personality disorder.
      6.2   Differentiate between psychodynamic and cognitive-behavioral explanations of this disorder and its treatment.

7.0   Schizoid Personality Disorder
      7.1   Describe the features of schizoid personality disorder and its relation to other schizophrenia spectrum disorders.
      7.2   Understand the limitations to treatment of this disorder.

8.0   Schizotypal Personality Disorder
      8.1   Indicate the features used to diagnose schizotypal personality disorder.
      8.2   Describe the relationship between schizophrenia and this personality disorder.

9.0   Avoidant Personality Disorder
      9.1   Explain the diagnostic features of avoidant personality disorder.
      9.2   Compare psychodynamic and cognitive-behavioral approaches to theory and treatment.

10.0   Dependent Personality Disorder
      10.1   Indicate the characteristics of dependent personality disorder.
      10.2   Differentiate between psychodynamic and cognitive-behavioral approaches to this disorder.

11.0   Obsessive-Compulsive Personality Disorder
      11.1   Describe the symptoms of obsessive-compulsive personality disorder.
      11.2   Contrast the psychodynamic and cognitive-behavioral perspectives.

12.0   Personality Disorders: The Biopsychosocial Perspective
      12.1   Comment on the challenges facing clinicians treating clients with personality disorders.

13.0   Chapter Boxes
      13.1   Discuss the case of author Susanna Kaysen.

Identifying the Disorder

Write the name of the personality disorder in the blank next to the symptoms listed.

1. _____ Lack of regard for the legal or moral standards of society. Some individuals with this disorder commit criminal or malicious acts..
2. _____ Unusual suspiciousness of others and constant attempts to guard oneself from harm.
3. _____ Eccentricities of thought, behavior, appearance, and ways of relating to others, often accompanied by peculiar beliefs.
4. _____ Chronic pattern of unstable mood, relationships, and identity.
5. _____ Excessive reliance on others, leading the individual to become incapable of making decisions or acting autonomously.
6. _____ Lack of interest in social relationships accompanied by emotional coldness and restrictiveness.
7. _____ Unrealistic, inflated sense of one's own importance.
8. _____ Overly dramatic emotionality in various realms of everyday behavior.
9. _____ Fear of closeness to others and being terrified by the prospect of being publicly embarrassed.
10._____ Unusual levels of perfectionism and rigidity.

Matching

Put the letter from the right-hand column corresponding to the correct match in the blank next to each item in the left-hand column.

1. ____ Exaggerated sense of self-importance seen in individuals with narcissistic personality disorder.
2. ____ Childhood disorder involving criminality that often precedes the development in adulthood of antisocial personality disorder.
3. ____ Term used to refer to the continuum of disorders including schizophrenia, schizotypal personality disorder, and schizoid personality disorder.
4. ____ The goal of treating antisocial personality disorder.
5. ____ Researcher who proposed that people with antisocial personality disorder are relatively insensitive to anxiety-provoking situations.
6. ____ Ability to restrain one's immediate urge to act; often lacking in children who later develop antisocial personality disorder.
7. ____ Term once used for schizotypal personality disorder.
8. ____ Therapeutic approach in which the clinician presents some harsh realities to a client.
9. ____ Suicidal gesture used to gain attention from others.
10. ____ Cognitive-behavioral theorist who developed a dialectical method of therapy for borderline personality.

a. confrontation
b. Marsha Linehan
c. impulse control
d. latent schizophrenia
e. stimulating feelings of remorse
f. grandiosity
g. conduct disorder
h. schizophrenia spectrum
i. Hervey Cleckley
j. Parasuicide

Short Answer

1. Contrast the psychodynamic and cognitive-behavioral explanations of each of the following personality disorders:

Personality disorder	Psychodynamic view	Cognitive-behavioral view
Borderline		
Paranoid		
Histrionic		
Narcissistic		
Avoidant		
Dependent		
Obsessive-compulsive		

2. Summarize the evidence for biological causes of the following personality disorders:

Disorder	Biological explanations
Antisocial personality disorder	
Borderline personality disorder	
Schizoid personality disorder	
Schizotypal personality disorder	

3. Answer the following questions concerning the nature of personality disorders, their diagnoses, and treatment.
    a. What is the difference between a personality trait and a personality disorder?

---

b. What factors do clinicians look for when diagnosing personality disorders?

_____

_____

c. What are two major problems involved in diagnosing these disorders?

_____

_____

d. How do clinicians attempt to set goals for treating clients with these disorders?

_____

_____

e. What is the role of a clinician's theoretical perspective in treating people with personality disorders?

_____

_____

4. For each of the following disorders, describe approaches to treatment and problems that are often encountered in implementing these treatments:

Disorder	Approach to treatment	Problems encountered in treatment
Antisocial personality disorder		
Borderline personality disorder		
Paranoid personality disorder		
Schizoid personality disorder		
Dependent personality disorder		
Obsessive-compulsive personality disorder		

5. Answer the following questions about brief psychodynamic treatment of personality disorders.

a. Why are clinicians attempting to develop shorter forms of therapy for personality disorders?

_____

_____

b. What specific techniques do clinicians use when doing brief therapy with personality disordered clients?

_____

_____

c. What does the research suggest about the effectiveness of time-limited or brief therapy for people with personality disorders?

_____

_____

d. Concerning the case of Harold Morrill, if Dr. Tobin were to use short-term therapy, what one theme or issue in his life do you think she might emphasize in order to maximize the benefits of their sessions?

_____

_____

From the Case Files of Dr. Sarah Tobin: Thinking About Harold's Case

Answer the following questions about the case of Harold Morrill.

1. What behaviors did Dr. Tobin observe during her first meeting with Harold that made her wary of her ability to work effectively with him?

_____

_____

_____

2. Briefly summarize the facts and conclusions that make up Dr. Tobin's formulation of Harold's case.

_____

_____

_____

3. What assessment instruments gave Dr. Tobin specific insight into the nature and extent of Harold's problems?

_____

_____

_____

4. Why was Dr. Tobin not surprised that her treatment plan was not successful with Harold?

_____

_____

_____

How <u>Are</u> We Different?

Answer the following questions about "How People Differ: Explaining the Prevalence of Borderline Personality Disorder among Women."

1. What behaviors associated with borderline personality disorder are stereotypically female?

    _____

    _____

2. What possible explanations (other than bias in the diagnostic criteria) are there to account for why more women than men are diagnosed with borderline personality disorder?

    _____

    _____

3. Referring to the discussion of the feminist-relational perspective of abnormality that was the subject of a text box in Chapter 4, comment on what contribution this perspective might make to explain the gender disparity between men and women who suffer from borderline personality disorder.

    _____

    _____

Review at a Glance

Test your knowledge by completing the blank spaces with terms from the chapter. If you need a hint, consult the chapter summary.

A (1)_____ involves a long lasting maladaptive pattern of inner experience and behavior, dating back to adolescence or young adulthood, that is manifested in at least two of the following areas: (2)_____, (3)_____, (4)_____, and (5)_____. This inflexible pattern is evident in various (6)_____ and (7)_____ situations, and cause (8)_____ or (9)_____. Personality disorders cause major (10)_____ and (11)_____ difficulty, leading to long-lasting impairment. The DSM-IV-TR separates personality disorders into three clusters based on shared characteristics. Cluster A comprises (12)_____, (13)_____, and (14)_____ personality disorders, which share the features of (15)_____ and (16)_____ behavior. Cluster B includes (17)_____, (18)_____, (19)_____, and (20)_____ personality disorders. People with these disorders are (21)_____, (22)_____, and (23)_____ or (24)_____. In Cluster C are (25)_____, (26)_____, and (27)_____ personality disorders, characterized by (28)_____ and (29)_____ behaviors.

People with (30)_____ have a lack of regard for society's moral or legal standards.

This diagnosis has its origins in Cleckley's notion of (31)_____, a personality type characterized by features such as (32)_____, (33)_____, (34)_____, (35)_____, and (36)_____. The *DSM-IV-TR* criteria added (37) _____ and (38) _____ behaviors. Biological theories suggest that this disorder has roots in (39) _____. Psychological theories focus on the notion that these individuals are unable to feel (40) _____ or_____ and to (41) _____. Sociocultural perspectives focus on (42) _____, (43)_____, and (44)_____ experiences. Experts recommend (45)_____ in treatment, especially in (46)_____ therapy.

Borderline personality disorder is characterized by (47) _____, (48) _____, and unstable (49) _____ and (50) _____. Many people with this condition engage in (51) _____ and (52) _____ behavior. Biological theory focuses on (53) _____ that may have evolved as a result of early (54) _____. Psychological theories have dwelled on (55) _____ and (56) _____ as predisposing factors. Sociocultural views focus on the possibility that many people develop this disorder as a result of (57) _____ in contemporary society. In terms of treatment, clinicians try to balance levels of (58) _____ and (59) _____, giving special attention to issues of (60) _____ and (61) _____. Linehan's (62) _____ involves components of (63) _____ and (64) _____.

(65)_____ personality disorder is characterized by excesses in emotionality and attention seeking. People with (66) _____personality disorder show a pattern of detachment from relationships and restricted range of emotional expression. Those with (67) _____ personality disorder show a pattern of social and interpersonal deficits marked by acute discomfort with and reduced capacity for close relationships. They also experience (68) _____ or _____ distortions and (69) _____. People with (70) _____ personality disorder show pervasive patterns of grandiosity, need for admiration, and lack of empathy. Avoidant personality disorder is characterized by a pattern of (71) _____, (72) _____, and (73) _____ to negative evaluation. People with (74) _____ personality disorder have an excessive need to be taken care of. The diagnosis of obsessive-compulsive personality disorder is characterized by a preoccupation with (75) _____, (76) _____, and (77) _____ and _____ control.

Given the lack of certainty about the causes of personality disorders, clinicians tend to focus on efforts to (78) _____ rather than attempt to bring about total change. Consequently, most

therapists (79) _____ treatment in response to the particular needs and difficulties of each

client.

Multiple Choice

1. Dr. Tobin noted Harold's turbulent relationships, unpredictable emotions, self-destructive behaviors, and identity disturbance and diagnosed him with which personality disorder?
   a. antisocial
   b. paranoid
   c. schizoid
   d. borderline

2. In treating people with antisocial personality disorder, it is recommended that the clinician
   a. adopt a confrontational approach.
   b. adopt a supportive approach.
   c. supplement psychotherapy with medication.
   d. bring the client's family into treatment.

3. Those who know Lisa have difficulty with her unpredictable vacillation between idealizing and devaluing other people, a symptom known as
   a. volatility.
   b. splitting.
   c. lability.
   d. ambivalence.

4. Psychodynamic explanations of paranoid personality disorder see it as rooted in the defense mechanism of
   a. rationalization.
   b. denial.
   c. projection.
   d. reaction formation.

5. Compared with people with avoidant personality disorder, those with schizoid personality disorder
   a. do not wish to have relationships.
   b. wish to have relationships.
   c. often suffer from a mood disorder.
   d. often are diagnosed with an Axis I disorder.

6. Researchers studying narcissistic and histrionic personality disorders have reported that
   a. the disorders can be easily differentiated.
   b. features of these two disorders overlap.
   c. both are genetically determined.
   d. they share the feature of hidden paranoia.

7. Cognitive-behavior theorists propose that people with obsessive-compulsive personality disorder
   a. have a hidden wish to be sloppy and disorderly.
   b. displace sexual energy into obsessional thinking and compulsive behavior.
   c. struggle with seemingly uncontrollable aggressive impulses.
   d. have their self-worth depend on conforming to an ideal abstract of perfectionism.

8. The higher prevalence of borderline personality disorder among women is explained by researchers as due to
   a. gender bias in the diagnostic criteria.
   b. disturbed family relationships.
   c. biological gender differences.
   d. higher sexual abuse during childhood.

9. A psychologist notes that a client's TAT stories are filled with themes of rage, intense feelings, identity confusion, and fears of abandonment. These themes correspond to which personality disorder?
   a. borderline
   b. antisocial
   c. schizotypal
   d. paranoid

10. When they were children, many adults who are diagnosed with antisocial personality disorder would have met the diagnostic criteria for
    a. dependent disorder.
    b. conduct disorder.
    c. antisocial disorder.
    d. histrionic disorder.

11. A core feature of people with narcissistic personality disorder is
    a. depression.
    b. mania.
    c. grandiosity.
    d. splitting.

160

12. Object relations theorists view people with dependent personality disorder as being
    a. insecurely attached.
    b. frustrated and hostile.
    c. self-defeating.
    d. passive-aggressive.

13. Diagnosis of a personality disorder is difficult because
    a. there may be a more specific problem for which the client seeks treatment.
    b. the disorders have such rigid diagnostic criteria.
    c. it is so difficult to detect the disorder in a person's behavior.
    d. these individuals are often aware that they have a problem but avoid seeking treatment.

14. A common developmental factor in the psychological environment of individuals with antisocial personality disorder is
    a. parental drug abuse.
    b. parental disharmony.
    c. abusive siblings.
    d. lack of schooling.

15. An inability to distinguish between one's own identity and the identities of others is characteristic of which personality disorder?
    a. schizoid
    b. self-defeating
    c. borderline
    d. narcissistic

16. In therapy, clients with borderline personality disorder are particularly likely to
    a. become aloof and distant from the therapist.
    b. describe their problems in vague and ambiguous terms.
    c. become pathologically dependent on the therapist.
    d. show narcissistic behavior.

17. It is difficult to treat people with schizoid and schizotypal personality disorder because
    a. they are emotionally unstable.
    b. they tend to view their therapist with suspicion.
    c. their treatment is often mandated by the courts.
    d. they are cognitively and emotionally out of touch.

18. According to current psychoanalytic theorists, parental failure to provide reassurance and positive responses to accomplishments may lead to the development of this personality disorder
    a. histrionic.
    b. schizoid.
    c. schizotypal.
    d. narcissistic.

19. Brief psychodynamic treatment of personality disorders is most likely to be effective when
    a. the client is resistant to establishing a working relationship.
    b. therapy takes an unfocused and global approach.
    c. there is a prominent interpersonal theme in the client's symptoms.
    d. the therapist avoids confrontation with the client on specific issues.

20. Which of the following is one of the most significant factors in determining whether or not an individual has a personality disorder?
    a. if they have trouble committing to relationships
    b. if they have been convicted of a crime related to their behavior
    c. if their problem has played a long-term role throughout their lives
    d. if they are having serious difficulty holding down a job

21. Which personality disorder is characterized by a lack of regard for society's moral and legal standards?
    a. antisocial
    b. borderline
    c. narcissistic
    d. passive-aggressive

22. Studies on family inheritance of criminal behavior have demonstrated that
    a. fraternal twins have a higher concordance rate for this type of behavior than do identical twins.
    b. sons are more likely to receive the extra Y chromosome from their mothers than from their fathers.
    c. identical twins have a higher concordance rate for this type of behavior than do fraternal twins.
    d. there is no set pattern that might indicate a genetic component.

23. The formation of intense and demanding relationships with others is characteristic of
    a. antisocial personality disorder.
    b. schizoid personality disorder.
    c. avoidant personality disorder.
    d. borderline personality disorder.

24. The personality disorder in which the primary symptom is constant efforts by the individual to attract attention with exaggerated displays of emotion is called
    a. histrionic personality disorder.
    b. borderline personality disorder.
    c. antisocial personality disorder.
    d. paranoid personality disorder.

25. Which personality disorder is characterized by an unrealistic, inflated sense of self-importance and an inability to see the perspectives of other people?
    a. borderline personality disorder
    b. obsessive-compulsive personality disorder
    c. passive-aggressive personality disorder
    d. narcissistic personality disorder

26. People with paranoid personality disorder tend to
    a. become overly dependent on others.
    b. engage in criminal acts.
    c. be impulsive.
    d. keep their distance from people.

27. What does the expression "schizophrenia spectrum disorders" mean?
    a. Schizophrenia, schizoid, and schizotypal personality disorders all involve visual hallucinations.
    b. Most of the personality disorders are related to schizophrenia.
    c. Borderline personality disorder is related to schizotypal personality disorder.
    d. Schizophrenia, schizoid, and schizotypal personality disorders may be on the same continuum.

28. Chris is a very shy 30-year-old woman who usually stays home and doesn't interact with other people. At work she strays away from the other people in the office as if she were afraid to talk to anyone. Chris might be diagnosed as suffering from
    a. avoidant personality disorder.
    b. antisocial personality disorder.
    c. dependent personality disorder.
    d. passive-aggressive personality disorder.

29. A serial killer would most likely be diagnosed with
    a. avoidant personality disorder
    b. dependent personality disorder
    c. histrionic personality disorder
    d. antisocial personality disorder

30. Lorraine always needs to be the center of attention. She talks loudly, gesturing wildly in hopes of gaining an audience. Everything in her life is, to hear her tell it, either far better or far worse than events in the lives of her friends. Lorraine may be suffering from
    a. dependent personality disorder
    b. histrionic personality disorder
    c. borderline personality disorder
    d. schizoid personality disorder

Answers

IDENTIFYING DISORDERS
1. antisocial
2. paranoid
3. schizotypal
4. borderline
5. dependent
6. schizoid
7. narcissistic
8. histrionic
9. avoidant
10. obsessive-compulsive

MATCHING
1. f
2. g
3. h
4. e
5. i
6. c
7. d
8. a
9. j
10. b

SHORT ANSWER
1.

Personality disorder	Psychodynamic view	Cognitive-behavioral view
Borderline	Problems in the early development of the self due to parents who either do not allow the child to achieve an independent identity or who are physically, emotionally, or sexually abusive.	Dichotomous thinking about the self and others and low sense of self-efficacy leading to lack of confidence, low motivation, and inability to seek long-term goals.
Paranoid	Heavy reliance on the defense mechanism of projection.	Mistaken assumptions that people will harm if they get the chance and that one needs to be wary of the malicious motives of others.
Histrionic	Traditional view is that histrionic personality disorder is a variant of hysteria, the product of unresolved Oedipal conflicts and overreliance on the defense mechanism of repression. Other psychoanalytic theorists propose that the disorder is the result of a global cognitive style that cannot focus on details in life situations.	Mistaken assumption that one is unable to handle life on one's own, causing the individual to seek someone else to make up for this deficit; the global nature of the individual's cognitive style leads to diffuse and exaggerated emotional states and unstable evaluations of others.
Narcissistic	Traditional explanation is that the disorder is due to failure to progress beyond early psychosexual stages of development. Object relations theorists propose that the individual develops the disorder in response to faulty parenting, in which the child is made to feel insecure and inadequate. This type of parenting leads the child to develop a false grandiose view of the self.	Faulty belief that one is special and deserves to be treated better than other people; problems result when these grandiose ideas about the self clash with experiences in the real world.

163

Personality disorder	Psychodynamic view	Cognitive-behavioral view
Avoidant	Horney's theory proposes that avoidant personality represents a "turning away from others" due to expectations that one will be criticized and rejected.	Hypersensitivity to rejection occurs due to childhood experiences of extreme criticism by parents. This leads to the faulty belief that one is flawed, unworthy, and undeserving of the attention and friendship of others. Avoidance develops as a means of protection from this anticipated rejection.
ependent	Traditional view is that the disorder reflects regression to or fixation at the oral stage of development due to overindulgence or neglect by parents of dependency needs. Object relations theorists view the disorder as the result of insecure attachment and low self-esteem.	Unassertiveness and anxiety over making independent decisions results from doubts about one's adequacy and ability to solve problems. Assertiveness with others would threaten the security of relationships.
Obsessive-compulsive	Traditional view is that the disorder is due to fixation at or regression to the anal stage of psychosexual development. More recent views emphasize an overly narrow and rigid cognitive style.	Unrealistic concern about being perfect and avoiding mistakes.

2.

Disorder	Biological explanations
Antisocial personality disorder	Extra chromosome (XYY pattern) Excess testosterone Defects in frontal lobes of cortex and/or limbic system Neuropsychological deficits in learning and attention Genetic inheritance
Borderline personality disorder	Genetic inheritance Abnormal neuroendocrine functions Electrophysiological functions
Schizoid personality disorder	Genetic inheritance possibly linked to schizophrenia.
Schizotypal personality disorder	Genetic inheritance possibly reflecting a latent form of schizophrenia.

3. a. A personality trait is an enduring pattern, as is a personality disorder, but a personality disorder is specifically identified as creating difficulties in the individual's life or feelings of personal distress.
    b. The clinician looks at the client's overall life history to determine whether the current problems have been present on a long-standing basis.
    c. The client often seeks treatment for other problems such as depression.
        Many personality disorders share similar features.
    d. Rather than seek complete personality change, clinicians tend to focus their work on achieving a set of more limited but realizable goals that will help alleviate the client's current distress.
    e. Most clinicians tend to individualize their treatment for the client's particular disorder and to integrate relevant theoretical perspectives that are most appropriate for the client's disorder.

4.

Disorder	Approach to treatment	Problems encountered in treatment
Antisocial personality disorder	Stimulate realization that client's behavior has caused harm to others. Reflect the selfish and self-defeating nature of the client's behavior.	Individuals with this disorder often do not seek help voluntarily and when in treatment, do not change easily.
Borderline personality disorder	Combine an approach that uses confrontation of client's maladaptive thoughts and defenses with providing a sense of stability and predictability. Help client recognize self-destructive nature of certain high-risk or harmful behaviors. Medication may also be used to alleviate symptoms of depression and anxiety.	Their volatility, inconsistency, and intensity make it difficult for these clients to remain in therapy. At the same time, clients may become pathologically dependent on their therapists.
Paranoid personality disorder	Cognitive-behavioral approach suggests countering client's mistaken assumptions and increasing client's self-efficacy. Generally, it is important to collaborate with client, increase client's awareness of other points of view, and help client become more assertive.	Client is likely to be distrustful of therapist and the therapy process.
Schizoid personality disorders	Help client clarify communication skills and modify isolated and eccentric behaviors.	Clients tend to be cognitively and emotionally inaccessible. Progress is likely to be slow and limited in scope.
Obsessive-compulsive personality disorder	Focus on client's maladaptive thoughts, possibly combining this approach with paradoxical instructions to become more symptomatic. Thought stopping techniques also applied.	Obsessive-compulsive client tends to ruminate excessively, and therapy might feed into this process.

5. a. Traditionally, therapies for people with personality disorders have been lengthy endeavors, often resulting in only limited change in their patterns of relating with others. Though not explicitly stated in the text box, insurance companies and managed care providers are also demanding short-term treatment.
   b. Steering the therapy sessions toward a central, maladaptive theme and confronting clients about styles of relating by calling attention to such behaviors as they arise in therapy; both are designed to heighten the client's emotional involvement in therapy.
   c. Research suggests that time-limited therapies are as effective as other forms of therapy, but even the typical "brief" therapy for personality disorders (6 to 12 months) is longer than brief therapy for other disorders.
   d. She would likely confront him about his manner of relating to her, his splitting (putting her on a pedestal at one point, criticizing her at another), and his problem with respecting the boundaries of therapy.

FROM THE CASE FILES OF DR. SARAH TOBIN: THINKING ABOUT HAROLD'S CASE

1. He idealized her, and he did not even know her. His appearance was unkempt and shaggy, and he looked immature for his age. He voiced intensity about his interactions with others, most of which ended in anger. He voiced no responsibility for any of the failures in his relationships.
2. The facts of Harold's past fit a pattern commonly seen in those with borderline personality disorder. His family was highly dysfunctional, his mother overprotective, and his father emotionally unavailable. His mother's control contributed to his inability to find a life for himself. He patterned his relationships after those of his parents. His mother's criticism left him with a lack of confidence about himself.

3. The WAIS-III subtest scores showed unevenness in his cognitive functioning. He showed deficits in comprehending tasks, yet he understood the issues. His MMPI-2 profile revealed serious personality disorganization with some psychotic-like features. His responses to the Rorschach test contained many unusual responses, with many references to sadistic human destruction, fire, and explosions. His TAT stories revealed themes of rage brought on by feelings of abandonment, characters were described as having sudden and chaotic mood changes, and his plots were disorganized.
4. Dr. Tobin has a lot of experience with borderline clients, with whom it is usually difficult to create and maintain a trusting therapeutic relationship. She was not surprised that her work with Harold came to an unsuccessful and frustrating end.

HOW ARE WE DIFFERENT?

1. Intensity of relationships and affective instability are stereotypical female traits.
2. Though differing biology (hormonal differences, sensitivity to endorphins) may play a role, history of sexual abuse appears to be a significant factor in the development of borderline personality disorder in girls (girls are more likely to be sexually abused than boys).
3. Inasmuch as women are more relationally oriented and more emotionally expressive, the feminist-relational approach would take that into account as a major factor in the development of borderline personality disorder in women whose childhoods are characterized by neglect, abuse, and trauma. Since relationships are so salient in the lives of most women, it stands to reason that their childhood experiences would leave them feeling frightened and insecure in their relations with others and would have provided a very bad model for their adult relationships.

REVIEW AT A GLANCE

1. personality disorder
2. cognition
3. affectivity
4. interpersonal functioning
5. impulse control
6. personal
7. social
8. distress
9. impairment
10. intrapsychic
11. interpersonal
12. paranoid
13. schizoid
14. schizotypal
15. odd
16. eccentric
17. antisocial
18. borderline
19. histrionic
20. narcissistic
21. overdramatic
22. emotional
23. erratic
24. unpredictable
25. avoidant
26. dependent
27. obsessive-compulsive
28. anxious
29. fearful
30. antisocial personality disorder
31. psychopathy
32. lack of remorse
33. extreme egocentricity
34. lack of emotional expressiveness
35. impulsivity
36. untruthfulness
37. disreputable
38. manipulative
39. brain abnormalities
40. fear or anxiety
41. process information not relevant to their immediate goals
42. family
43. early environment
44. socialization
45. confrontation
46. group
47. poor impulse control
48. fluctuating self-image
49. mood
50. interpersonal relationships
51. splitting
52. parasuicidal
53. brain differences
54. trauma
55. trauma
56. abuse
57. diminished cohesion
58. support
59. confrontation
60. stability
61. boundaries
62. dialectical behavior therapy
63. acceptance
64. confrontation
65. Histrionic
66. schizoid
67. schizotypal
68. cognitive; perceptual distortions
69. behavioral eccentricities
70. narcissistic
71. social inhibition
72. feelings of inadequacy
73. hypersensitivity
74. dependent
75. orderliness
76. perfectionism
77. mental; interpersonal
78. improve the client's current life experiences

79. individualize

MULTIPLE CHOICE
1. (d) is correct. (a), (b), and (c) are not characterized by the described behaviors.
2. (a) is correct. (b), (c), and (d) would not be effective techniques for an antisocial client.
3. (b) is correct. (a), (c), and (d) do not characterize moving from devaluation to idealization.
4. (c) is correct. (a), (b), and (d) do not typify a paranoid personality.
5. (a) is correct. (b) is true of those with avoidant disorder; there is no reason to expect that (c) and (d) would be true.
6. (b) is correct. (a), (c) , and (d) are not correct statements.
7. (d) is correct. There is no evidence that (a), (b), and (c) would be correct statements.
8. (d) is correct. There is no evidence that (a) and (c) are relevant; (b) is a fact in many homes.
9. (a) is correct. (b), (c), and (d) are not characterized by the described behaviors.
10. (b) is correct. (a) and (d) are not related to antisocial disorder and (c) is not diagnosed before the age of 18.
11. (c) is correct. (a), (b), and (d) are not associated with narcissistic personality disorder.
12. (a) is correct. (b), (c), and (d) are not associated with dependent personality disorder.
13. (a) is correct. (b), (c), and (d) are not true. In fact the opposite of these statements is more likely.
14. (b) is correct. (a), (c), and (d) are not known to be related to the development of antisocial personality disorder.
15. (c) is correct. (a), (b), and (d) are not characterized by this problem with boundaries.
16. (c) is correct. (a), (b), and (c) would not be behaviors expected of a borderline client. . (a) is not correct although it comes close to the idea of splitting where the client will become dependent on the therapist (c) and other times become angry at them
17. (d) is correct. (a), (b), or (c) would not necessarily characterize these clients. Schizotypal personalities express some suspiciousness towards others (b) but schizoid personalities do not.
18. (d) is correct. This factor is not generally related to the development of (a), (b), or (c).
19. (c) is correct. (a), (b), and (d) would make it likely that brief therapy would not be successful.
20. (c) is correct. (a), (b), and (d) may be indicated in several types of disorders, not just personality disorders. (a) may relate to specific types of personality disorders such as borderline, schizoid, and avoidant personality disorders.
21. (a) is correct. (b), (c), and (d) are not associated with the described behaviors.
22. (c) is correct. (a), (b), and (d) are not supported by current research.
23. (d) is correct. (b) and (c) would be unlikely to form intense relationships; relationship style has not been a focus of study with (a).
24. (a) is correct. (b), (c), and (d) are not characterized by this type of behavior.
25. (d) is correct. (a), (b), and (c) are not typified by this behavior.
26. (d) is correct. (a) is the virtual opposite of (d); (b) and (c) are not consistent with paranoid personality disorder.
27. (d) is correct. There is no basis for the statements in (a), (b), and (c).
28. (a) is correct. The behaviors described are not associated with (b), (c), or (d).
29. (d) is correct. The behaviors described are not associated with (b), (c), or (d).
30. (b) is correct. The behaviors described are not associated with (a), (c), or (d).

CHAPTER 11
DEVELOPMENT-RELATED DISORDERS

CHAPTER AT A GLANCE

Development-Related Disorders

Mental Retardation
Characteristics
Theories and Treatment

Pervasive Developmental Disorders
Characteristics
Theories and Treatment

Learning, Communication and Motor Skills Disorders
Characteristics
Theories and Treatment

Separation Anxiety Disorder
Characteristics
Theories and Treatment

Attention Deficit and Disruptive Behavior Disorders
ADHD
Conduct Disorder
Oppositional Defiant Disorder
Theories and Treatment

Other Disorders that Originate in Childhood
Childhood Eating Disorders
Tic Disorders
Elimination Disorders
Reactive Attachment Disorder
Stereotypic Movement Disorder
Selective Mutism

Learning Objectives

1.0   Introductory Issues
    1.1   Discuss the controversies involved in the definition and diagnosis of development-related disorders.

2.0   Mental Retardation
    2.1   Identify the characteristics of mental retardation and the behavioral competencies associated with the different levels of retardation.
    2.2   Describe the causes of mental retardation including the genetic and environmental factors and prevention programs.
    2.3   Discuss the treatments and interventions best suited for people with mental retardation.

3.0   Pervasive Developmental Disorders
    3.1   Identify the types and characteristics of pervasive developmental disorders, including Rett's disorder, childhood disintegrative disorder, and Asperger's disorder.
    3.2   Describe the characteristics of autistic disorder and those of its subtype, autistic savant syndrome.
    3.3   Summarize current explanations of autistic disorder, psychopharmacological and behavioral treatments of autistic disorder, and the controversies associated with aversive treatment techniques.

4.0   Learning, Communication, and Motor Skills Disorders
    4.1   Identify the characteristics of learning disorders.
    4.2   Indicate the diagnostic features of communication disorders.
    4.3   Describe the symptoms of motor skills disorders.
    4.4   Summarize current theories and treatments of learning, communication, and motor skills disorders.

5.0   Attention Deficit and Disruptive Behavior Disorders
    5.1   Identify the characteristics of attention-deficit hyperactivity disorder.
    5.2   Describe the symptoms of conduct disorder.
    5.3   Indicate the diagnostic features of oppositional-defiant disorder.
    5.4   Discuss the theories and treatments of ADHD and disruptive behavior disorders.

6.0   Separation Anxiety Disorders
    6.1   Indicate the symptoms of separation anxiety disorder.
    6.2   Evaluate the theories and treatment of separation anxiety disorder.

7.0   Other Disorders that Originate in Childhood
    7.1   Describe the features of childhood eating disorders.
    7.2   Indicate the nature of tic disorders.
    7.3   Summarize the characteristics of elimination disorders.
    7.4   Identify the symptoms of reactive attachment disorder.
    7.5   Describe the diagnostic criteria for stereotypic movement disorder.
    7.6   Indicate the features of selective mutism.

8.0   Development-Related Disorders: The Biopsychosocial Perspective

9.0   Chapter Boxes
    9.1   Discuss aspects of the case of Edward Hallowell.
    9.2   Identify advances in the treatment of ADHD.

Identifying Symptoms

Write the name of the disorder in which the symptom described is a prominent feature.

1. _____ Delay or deficit in a particular academic skill.
2. _____ Refusal to talk when a social interaction is expected.
3. _____ Impulsive, restless, aggressive, and unable to focus on a task.
4. _____ Significantly below-average intellectual functioning and adaptive behavior.
5. _____ Involved in delinquent and criminal activities without remorse for one's actions.
6. _____ Massive impairment in ability to communicate and relate emotionally to others.
7. _____ Hostile, argumentative, and generally rebellious toward authority figures.
8. _____ Distress when parents are not present even for short periods of time.
9. _____ Severely handicapped communication and emotional relatedness combined with extraordinary skill in an area such as memory or arithmetic.
10. _____ Repetitive, seemingly driven bodily behaviors that interfere with everyday functioning and can cause injuries.
11. _____ In females, impaired cognitive and neurological development between 5 months and 4 years of age.
12. _____ Difficulty understanding and expressing certain kinds of words or phrases.
13. _____ Normal development for first 2 years with loss of cognitive and adaptive skills before the age of 10.
14. _____ Obvious problems of verbal expression.
15. _____ Adequate cognitive and language development with severe impairment in social interaction and restricted, repetitive, and stereotyped patterns of behavior.

Matching

Put the letter from the right-hand column corresponding to the correct match in the blank next to each item in the left-hand column.

1. ___ Abnormalities in this neurotransmitter system are thought to be a source of attention-deficit/hyperactivity disorder.
2. ___ Level of mental retardation in which individual can be trained but is unlikely to progress beyond second-grade skills.
3. ___ Disorder in which child regurgitates food after it has been swallowed, possibly eating the vomit after it has been spit up.
4. ___ Speech and language disorder characterized by mispronunciations, substitutions, and omissions of speech sounds.
5. ___ Form of mental retardation caused by chromosomal abnormality present from conception.
6. ___ Disorder of childhood in which child lacks control of bowel movements.
7. ___ In developmental _____ disorder, an individual has difficulty performing simple physical tasks.
8. ___ Medication found to be helpful in reducing symptoms of attention-deficit/hyperactivity disorder.
9. ___ Childhood disorder involving recurrent eating of inedible substances such as hair, paper, and string.
10. ___ Approach that is mandated by U.S. federal law to integrate children with mental retardation into public schools.
11. ___ Level of retardation in which an individual can respond to a very limited range of self-help training.
12. ___ A tic disorder that involves involuntary uttering of obscenities.
13. ___ Form of pervasive developmental disorder shown by the title character in *Rain Man*, who could instantly make complex math calculations.
14. ___ Speech and language disorder characterized by limited vocabulary and use of grammatical structures.
15. ___ Disorder in which child lacks control over urination.

a. mainstreaming
b. pica
c. Tourette's syndrome
d. coordination
e. catecholamine
f. encopresis
g. moderate
h. expressive language disorder
i. autistic savant syndrome
j. enuresis
k. Down syndrome
l. rumination disorder
m. methylphenidate
n. phonological disorder
o. profound

Short Answer

1. In what ways are the following pairs of items the same?

a. Tay-Sachs disease and Fragile X syndrome: _____
b. Phonological disorder and receptive language disorder: _____
c. Echolalia and emotional unresponsiveness: _____
d. Pica and ruminative disorder: _____
e. Mathematics disorder and disorder of written expression: _____
f. White noise and cold showers: _____
g. Oppositional defiant disorder and conduct disorder: _____

h. Albert Einstein and Henry Ford: _____

i. Facial abnormalities and low birth weight: _____

2. Describe the possible role of biological factors as causes of each of the following development-related disorders:

Development-related disorder	Possible biological factors
Mental retardation	
Autistic disorder	
Language, communication, and motor skills disorders	
Attention-deficit/hyperactivity disorder	
Separation anxiety disorder	

3. Summarize long-term effects associated with each of the following disorders:

Disorder	Long-term effects
Autistic disorder	
Language, communication, and motor skills disorders	
Conduct disorder	
Attention-deficit/hyperactivity disorder	
Separation anxiety disorder	

4. Imagine that you are a parent of a child with attention-deficit/hyperactivity disorder. List three advantages and three disadvantages that you would consider if choosing medication such as Ritalin (methylphenidate) as a method of treatment?

Advantages	Disadvantages

5. Briefly describe the available behavioral treatments for each of the following development-related disorders:

Disorder	Behavioral treatment
Mental retardation	
Autistic disorder	
Learning, communication, and motor skills disorders	
Attention-deficit/hyperactivity disorder	
Conduct disorder	
Separation anxiety disorder	

ABC Puzzle

Fill in each of the following blanks that are in alphabetical order. The first letter of the answer is indicated at the beginning of the blank:

A _____ Disorder involving massive deficits in a person's ability to communicate and form emotional bonds with others.

B _____ Theoretical perspective on which aversive conditioning procedures are based.

C _____ Disorder in which a child becomes involved in criminal or delinquent activities and feels no sense of remorse.

D _____ Category of disorders that applies specifically to children.

E _____ Characteristic of autistic disorder in which the individual repetitively utters the sound of a verbalization.

F _____ Cause of mental retardation due to an abnormality on the "X" chromosome.

G _____ Category of causes of mental retardation due to deficits or abnormalities in a person's inherited potential.

H _____ Common term for a child who is incapable of sustaining attention on a task, becomes restless, and can irritate others by constant movement and aggressiveness.

I   _____   Psychological variable on which categories of mental retardation are based.

J   _____   Religious/ethnic background of people who are most vulnerable to inheriting Tay-Sachs disease.

K   _____   Expert on autistic disorder who theorized that faulty mothering is the cause of the disorder.

L   _____   Disorders involving delays or deficits in acquiring academic skills

M   _____   Disorder in which individual suffers delays or deficits in acts involving coordination.

N   _____   Historically renowned physicist who was a poor student in school and a failure in running the family farm.

O   _____   Form of disruptive behavior disorder characterized by extreme stubbornness, rebelliousness, and resistance to authority.

P   _____   Mental retardation caused by failure (present at birth) to produce an enzyme needed for normal development.

Q   _____   A child with selective mutism is very _____ because he or she refuses to speak.

R   _____   Commonly known as "German measles," a disease that can cause mental retardation if the mother acquires it during the first trimester of pregnancy.

S   _____   Disorder in which the individual shows a disturbance in the normal fluency and patterning of speech.

T   _____   Rapid, recurring, involuntary movement or vocalization.

U   _____   Environmental cause of mental retardation that is associated with high poverty levels and poor diets.

V   _____   Patterns of rising crime and _____ are seen as contributing to behavioral problems among inner-city youth.

W   _____   Use of these on cigarette boxes and alcohol labels is regarded as aiding in prevention of mental retardation.

X   _____   Computer-aided versions of this radiological test can provide important information about brain abnormalities in people with disorders such as autistic disorder.

Y   _____   Synonym for childhood and adolescence.

Z   _____   Snoring noise made by weary students.

Focusing on Research

Answer the following questions from "Research Focus: Advances in Treatment of ADHD":

1. What were the results of the MTA study?

_____

_____

2. What was the role of parental involvement in mediating symptom improvement?

_____

_____

From the Case Files of Dr. Sarah Tobin: Thinking About Jason's Case

Answer the following questions about the case of Jason Newman.

1. Describe Dr. Tobin's observations of Jason at their first meeting.

    _____

    _____

2. List Jason's symptoms as reported by his parents.

    _____

    _____

3. Identify the components of Dr. Tobin's assessment of Jason and her diagnosis.

    _____

    _____

4. Discuss the nature and course of Jason's treatment.

    _____

    _____

Review at a Glance

Test your knowledge by completing the blank spaces with terms from the chapter. If you need a hint, consult the chapter summary.

An IQ of (1) _____ or below indicates mental retardation. In addition to intellectual deficits, people with mental retardation have significant impairments in abilities such as (2) _____, (3) _____, (4) _____, and (5) _____. Mental retardation can result from and (6) _____ condition or from an (7) _____ or _____ that takes place during development.

(8) _____ disorders are characterized by severe impairment in (9) _____, (10) _____ skills, or the presence of extremely odd (11) _____, (12) _____, and (13) _____. The most common of these disorders is (14) _____ disorder, characterized by massive impairment in an individual's ability to (15) _____ and relate (16) _____ to others. Support for the biological theory of autism includes patterns of (17) _____, as well as studies of brain (18) _____ and (19) _____. Psychological interventions aim at modifying the (20) _____ of autistic individuals.

A (21) _____ is a delay or deficit in (22) _____ that is evident when an individual's achievement on standardized tests is (23) _____ what would be expected for others of comparable (24) _____, (25) _____, and level of (26) _____. (27) _____ are characterized by impairment in the (28) _____ or (29) _____ of language. The primary form of (30) _____ disorder is (31)

_____, a condition characterized by marked impairment in the development of (32) _____. Most developmental disorders are viewed as (33) _____ based, with various causes, such as damage during (34) _____ or (35) _____ or as the result of (36) _____ or a (37) _____. Interventions for children with these disorders generally occur in a (38) _____ setting.

Attention-deficit/hyperactivity disorder (ADHD) involves (39) _____ and (40) _____. Inattentiveness is characterized by behaviors such as (41) _____, forgetfulness in (42) _____, and other (43) _____ problems. The hyperactive-impulsive component is further divided into subtypes of (44) _____ and (45) _____. Hyperactivity is characterized by (46) _____, (47) _____, (48) _____ inappropriately, having difficulty in (49) _____ quietly, and (50) _____ excessively. Impulsivity is evident in individuals who (51) _____, (52) _____, and (53) _____ or _____ on others. Young people with (54) _____ persistently (55) _____, while those with oppositional defiant disorder show a pattern of (56) _____, (57) _____, and (58) _____ behaviors that result in (59) _____ or _____ problems.

Extensive research on the causes of ADHD focuses on (60) _____ abnormality that accounts for impaired (61) _____ and (62) _____. The most common biological intervention is the medication (63) _____. Psychological interventions are based on (64) _____ principles.

(65)_____ involves the experience of intense and inappropriate anxiety concerning separation from (66) _____ or _____. Childhood eating disorders include conditions such as (67) _____, (68) _____ of infancy or early childhood, and (69) _____ disorder. Tic disorders, such as (70) _____ disorder, involve bodily (71) _____ or (72) _____. Elimination disorders, such as (73) _____ and (74) _____, are characterized by failure to maintain continence at an age-appropriate stage. (75)_____ is a severe disturbance in an individual's ability to relate to others. Individuals with (76) _____ disorders engage in repetitive, seemingly driven bodily movements. Those with (77) _____ refuse to talk in certain circumstances.

Multiple Choice

1. Researchers studying adults with ADHD have found that many experience
   a. other serious psychological disorders.
   b. higher than average intelligence.
   c. improved psychological adjustment.
   d. lower cognitive distractibility.

2. A form of mental retardation with brain changes similar to those found in Alzheimer's disease is
   a. Fragile X syndrome.
   b. Tay-Sachs disease.
   c. phenylketonuria.
   d. Down syndrome.

3. The most appropriate intervention for an individual diagnosed with PKU is
   a. exposure to full-spectrum light.
   b. a special diet.
   c. low dose radiation.
   d. neuroleptic medication.

4. Which of the following is a procedure that is used to detect chromosomal abnormalities in a developing fetus?
   a. amniocentesis
   b. chromosonography
   c. genetic mapping
   d. FAS screening

5. Mainstreaming is
   a. the establishment of institutions that are devoted to educating people with disabilities.
   b. the placement of children with disabilities in foster homes where they can be appropriately nurtured.
   c. the integration into society of people with mental and physical disabilities.
   d. legislation that requires alcohol and tobacco products to carry warnings about potential toxic effects.

6. Which of the following is characteristic of Asperger's disorder?
   a. normal cognitive and language development
   b. occurrence only in females
   c. severe social and motor impairments
   d. loss of adaptive functions after the age of 10 years

7. Eleven-year-old Jonah's speech is characterized by poor use of grammar and vocabulary relative to others of his age, although he is able to understand the speech of others. These are signs that he has which communication disorder?
   a. stuttering
   b. expressive language disorder
   c. phonological disorder
   d. mixed receptive-expressive language disorder

8. Michael is a third-grader who is often causing problems at home and school. He is disorganized, messy, impulsive, inattentive, and accident-prone. In all likelihood, Michael would be regarded as having
   a. attention-deficit/hyperactivity disorder.
   b. conduct disorder.
   c. oppositional defiant disorder.
   d. separation anxiety disorder.

9. Which disorder is diagnosed in children who have great difficulty relating to others and express this either in avoidance of social interactions or in inappropriate familiarity with strangers?
   a. selective mutism
   b. separation anxiety disorder
   c. atypical autistic disorder
   d. reactive attachment disorder

10. In what context is a restrained time-out station used?
    a. aversive treatment for individuals with autistic disorder
    b. positive reinforcement for individuals with learning disorders
    c. behavioral treatment of hyperactive children
    d. rehabilitation of mentally retarded individuals

11. In explaining the hypothesized causes of ADHD, experts currently believe that it
    a. develops as a result of inadequate intellectual stimulation.
    b. is a genetically acquired trait.
    c. develops primarily as a result of a disturbed family system.
    d. is biologically based, triggered by certain stressful environmental conditions.

12. The term used to describe behavior in which an individual has bowel movements in clothes or inappropriate places is
    a. encopresis.
    b. enuresis.
    c. dyslexia.
    d. coprolalia.

13. The metabolic disorder that causes neural degeneration and early death, usually before the child reaches the age of 4 is called
    a. Down syndrome.
    b. Fragile X syndrome.
    c. phenylketonuria.
    d. Tay-Sachs syndrome.

14. A syndrome involving mental retardation that develops in the child of a woman who regularly consumes excess amounts of liquor while she is pregnant is referred to as
    a. Fragile X syndrome.
    b. alcohol dependence syndrome.
    c. Tay-Sachs syndrome.
    d. fetal alcohol syndrome.

15. Autistic children usually form attachments to
    a. inanimate objects.
    b. pets.
    c. older siblings.
    d. their mothers.

16. MRI scans of the brains of individuals with autistic disorder reveal
    a. temporal lobe malformations.
    b. low levels of cortical arousal.
    c. enlarged ventricles.
    d. lesions in the hypothalamus.

17. Norm has just started 1st grade but does not understand what his teacher means when she asks him to count to 10. He is also baffled by her requests to add or subtract numbers. Norm might be diagnosed as having
    a. math phobia.
    b. mathematics disorder.
    c. expressive numeric disorder.
    d. dyscalcula.

18. Which of the following is the development-related disorder that is the precursor in childhood of antisocial personality disorder?
    a. overanxious disorder
    b. conduct disorder
    c. oppositional defiant disorder
    d. attention-deficit/hyperactivity disorder

19. In many ways, Sally seems like a typical teenager. However, she repeatedly argues with her parents, refuses to do what she is told, and at times does things to annoy people deliberately. If this behavior pattern is relatively long-term, Sally might have
    a. conduct disorder.
    b. attention-deficit/hyperactivity disorder.
    c. rumination disorder.
    d. oppositional defiant disorder.

20. Seth is constantly moving his head and twitching his shoulders. He utters loud, abrupt noises that others regard as strange. These movement and vocal patterns are uncontrollable. The term used to describe Seth's condition is
    a. Rett syndrome.
    b. Sack's disorder.
    c. Asperger's syndrome.
    d. Tourette's disorder.

21. In order to be considered mentally retarded, an individual's IQ must be
    a. between 100-120.
    b. between 80-100.
    c. between 75-80.
    d. less than 70.

22. A condition caused by poverty and neglect in which the child does not grow at a normal rate either physically or mentally is known as
    a. failure to thrive.
    b. anoxia.
    c. retardation.
    d. Tay-Sachs disease.

23. A symptom of autistic disorder in which the child mimics other people's words or phrases is referred to as
    a. clanging.
    b. perseveration.
    c. reverberating.
    d. echolalia.

24. Joshua has a specific developmental disorder that is characterized by the fact that words and letters get reversed when he is reading; for example, the letter "b" looks like "d" and the word "frog" may look like "gorf." This problem makes him read aloud in a slow and broken way. Joshua may have
    a. disorder of written expression.
    b. cluttering.
    c. expressive language disorder.
    d. dyslexia.

25. Which disorders may be the result of difficulty integrating information from the brain areas involved in vision, speech, and language comprehension?
    a. disruptive behavior disorders
    b. learning, communication, and motor skills disorders
    c. anxiety disorders of childhood
    d. pervasive developmental disorders

26. Victor generally has no difficulty sitting still but cannot focus his attention on what the teacher is saying for long periods of time. Victor might be diagnosed as having
    a. attention-deficit/hyperactivity disorder, inattentive type.
    b. attention-deficit/hyperactivity disorder, hyperactive-impulsive type.
    c. attention-deficit/hyperactivity disorder, combined type.
    d. attention-deficit/hyperactivity disorder, overactive type.

27. While eating, Lindsay often spits her food back up and rechews it. Assuming that this is a persistent problem, Lindsay might be diagnosed with
    a. pica
    b. feeding disorder of early childhood
    c. rumination disorder
    d. bulimia nervosa

28. The disorder originating in childhood in which the individual voluntarily repeats nonproductive behaviors such as rocking or head banging is called
    a. elective mutism.
    b. childhood schizophrenia.
    c. stereotypic movement disorder.
    d. pica.

Answers

IDENTIFYING SYMPTOMS

1. learning disorder
2. selective mutism
3. attention-deficit/hyperactivity disorder
4. mental retardation
5. conduct disorder
6. autistic disorder
7. oppositional defiant disorder
8. separation anxiety disorder
9. autistic savant syndrome
10. stereotypic movement disorder
11. Rett's disorder
12. mixed receptive-expressive language disorder
13. childhood disintegrative disorder
14. expressive language disorder
15. Asperger's disorder

MATCHING

1. e
2. g
3. l
4. n
5. k
6. f
7. d
8. m
9. b
10. a
11. o
12. c
13. i
14. h
15. j

SHORT ANSWER

1. a. Causes of mental retardation
   b. Communication disorders
   c. Symptoms of autistic disorder
   d. Eating disorders of childhood
   e. Learning disorders
   f. Aversive treatments for autistic disorder
   g. Disruptive behavior disorders
   h. Successful adults who had learning problems in school
   i. Characteristics of children born with fetal alcohol syndrome

2.

Development-related disorder	Possible biological factors
Mental retardation	Mental retardation can be due to an inherited inability to utilize phenylalanin (PKU), disrupted metabolism (Tay-Sachs disease), sex chromosome abnormalities (Fragile X Syndrome), chromosomal aberrations during conception (Down Syndrome), or rubella contracted by the mother during the first trimester of pregnancy.
Autistic disorder	People with autistic disorder show abnormal EEGs, CAT scans, and MRIs as well as serotonin abnormalities.
Language, communication, and motor skills disorders	Damage to various brain sites during fetal development, birth, or early childhood.

Attention-deficit/hyperactivity disorder	Evidence for the heritability of ADHD is among the highest rates for all psychiatric disorders and probably involves several genes related to dopamine. There also tend to be smaller volumes in frontal cortex, cerebellum, and subcortical structures.
Separation anxiety disorder	Separation anxiety in children related to increased panic disorder in parents, suggesting a possible genetic link.

3.

Disorder	Long-term effects
Autistic disorder	Two-thirds of people with autistic disorder are unable to live an independent life as an adult.
Language, communication, and motor skills disorders	Increased risk of anxiety disorder, mood disorder, ADHD, conduct disorder, and adjustment disorder.
Conduct disorder	Marital difficulties, decreased occupational and educational opportunities, poor social relationships, alcohol use, poorer physical health, and antisocial personality disorder as adults.
Attention-deficit hyperactivity disorder	Relationship problems, academic problems, depression,
Separation anxiety disorder	Increased likelihood of developing anxiety disorder as an adult.

4.

Advantages	Disadvantages
Increased attentional control	Decreased sleep
Decreased hyperactive behavior	Decreased appetite
Increased positive social interactions with peers, teachers, and parents	Development of twitches

5.

Disorder	Behavioral treatment
Mental retardation	Reinforcement for appropriate use of speech and language, and the development of social skills; parents can be taught to reward a child for appropriate behaviors and to respond negatively to inappropriate behaviors.
Autistic disorder	Self-control procedures, relaxation training, covert conditioning, and in extreme cases, aversive therapy.
Learning, communication, and motor skills disorders	In the school context, more structure, fewer distractions, presentation of new material that uses more than one sensory modality at a time.
Attention-deficit/hyperactivity disorder	Psychoeducation, instilling hope and optimism, compensatory behavioral/self-management training, marital counseling, family therapy, career counseling, group therapy, college planning, coaching focusing on goals, computer programs or personal digital assistants, school and/or workplace accommodations that facilitate productivity and minimize distraction, teaching self-advocacy..
Conduct disorder	Teach appropriate behaviors such as cooperation and self-control while unlearning problem behaviors such as aggression, stealing, and lying; use reinforcement, behavioral contracting, modeling, and relaxation training.
Separation anxiety disorder	Systematic desensitization, prolonged exposure, and modeling; contingency management and self-management can also teach the child to react more competently to a fear-provoking situation.

ABC PUZZLE

Autistic disorder	Jewish	Stuttering
Behavioral	Kanner	Tic
Conduct disorder	Learning disorders	Undernutrition
Development-related disorders	Motor skills disorder	Violence
Echolalia	Newton (Sir Isaac)	Warning labels
Fragile X	Oppositional defiant disorder	X-rays
Genetic	Phenylketonuria	Youth
Hyperactive	Quiet	Z-Z-Z (Sorry, we couldn't find
Intelligence	Rubella	any "z" words in this chapter!)

FOCUSING ON RESEARCH

1. Medication, and medication + psychotherapy were more effective than behavioral or community care in reducing the symptoms of ADHD.
2. Parental attitudes and disciplinary practices played a crucial role in mediating symptom improvement.

FROM THE CASE FILES OF DR. SARAH TOBIN: THINKING ABOUT JASON'S CASE

1. Jason had just knocked over a water cooler causing water to go all over the floor. While Jason's mother scolded him, Jason played a game on his handheld Nintendo. He made popping noises with his mouth and cheered his game results. When Dr. Tobin met with Jason alone, he ignored some of her questions, changed topics, interrupted her, and was constantly distracted.
2. He was unable to control his behavior, was antagonizing people at home and other children at school, out of control at home and school, recently set a fire at school, disrupting his classes at school, throwing things at other students, playing tricks on his teachers, refusing to wait his turn, unable to sit still at church, at a movie, or during dinner at home, and was not paying attention in school, or doing his homework.
3. He had recently had an IQ test at school which placed him in the above-average range of intelligence on verbal and performance scales. Dr. Tobin had Jason's parents and teachers complete the Connors Checklist of Child Behaviors. The results indicated learning problems, impulsivity, and hyperactivity. She diagnosed Jason with ADHD combined type.
4. Jason started taking Ritalin and participated in individual therapy with a child psychiatrist, weekly for six months, then monthly thereafter. His parents were trained in a behavioral management program. He did not improve overnight, but he improved steadily. His parents were successful in following the home behavioral management plan.

REVIEW AT A GLANCE

1. 70
2. social skills
3. judgment
4. communication
5. self-care
6. inherited
7. event; illness
8. Pervasive developmental
9. social interaction
10. communication
11. behaviors
12. interests
13. activities
14. autistic
15. communicate
16. emotionally
17. familial inheritance
18. size
19. structure
20. maladaptive behaviors
21. learning disorder
22. academic skill
23. substantially below
24. age
25. education
26. intelligence
27. Communication disorders
28. expression
29. understanding
30. motor skills
31. developmental coordination disorder
32. motor coordination

33. neurologically
34. fetal development
35. birth
36. physical trauma
37. medical disorder
38. school
39. inattentiveness
40. hyperactivity-impulsivity
41. carelessness
42. daily activities
43. attentional
44. hyperactivity
45. impulsivity
46. fidgeting
47. being restless
48. running about

49. playing
50. talking
51. blurt out answers
52. cannot wait their turn
53. interrupt; intrude
54. conduct disorder
55. violate the rights of others
56. negativistic
57. hostile
58. defiant
59. family; school
60. neurological
61. behavioral inhibition
62. self-control
63. methylphenidate (Ritalin)
64. behavioral

65. Separation anxiety disorder
66. home; caregivers
67. pica
68. feeding disorder
69. rumination disorder
70. Tourette's
71. movement
72. vocalizations
73. encopresis
74. enuresis
75. Reactive attachment
    disorder
76. stereotypic movement
77. selective mutism

MULTIPLE CHOICE

1. (a) is correct. ADHD has not been found to be related to (b), (c), or (d).
2. (d) is correct. (a), (b), and (c) are dissimilar to Alzheimer's disease.
3. (b) is correct. (a), (c), and (d) are not used to treat PKU.
4. (a) is correct. There is no such procedure as (b); (c) is not a diagnostic procedure; (d) screens for fetal alcohol syndrome.
5. (c) is correct. (a) and (b) are antithetical to (c); (d) has nothing to do with integration of the disabled into society.
6. (c) is correct. (a), (b), and (d) are not associated with Asperger's disorder.
7. (b) is correct. (a) is an expressive disorder; in which the fluency of speech is interrupted; (c) is another expressive disorder in which the child cannot articulate the appropriate sounds; and (d) is a combination of both types of receptive and expressive disorders.
8. (a) is correct. The described behaviors are not associated with (b), (c), or (d).
9. (d) is correct. (a) is a refusal to speak; (b) involves anxiety when separated from caregivers; and (c) is a pervasive developmental disorder.
10. (c) is correct. (a), (b), and (d) are not reasons for a restrained time-out.
11. (d) is correct. (a), (b), and (c) are not known to be related to ADHD.
12. (a) is correct. (b) involves urination; (c) is a reading disorder; (d) is a speech disorder.
13. (d) is correct. (a) and (b) do not result in early death; (c) will not result in death if a standard treatment regimen is followed.
14. (d) is correct. (a) may be related to mental retardation, but not as the result of a mother's alcohol consumption; (c) is not related to alcohol; and (b) is not related to mental retardation.
15. (a) is correct. They usually are not as interested in (b), (c), or (d).
16. (c) is correct. There is not research evidence for (a), (b), or (d).
17. (b) is correct. (a) and (c) are not disorders; (d) is related to numbers, but does not fit the described example.
18. (b) is correct. (a) is not a disorder; (c) involves defiance of authority; (d) is an attentional disorder.
19. (d) is correct. (a) involves behaviors violating of the rights of others; (b) is an attentional disorder; and (c) is an eating disorder.
20. (d) is correct. (c) is a pervasive developmental disorder ; (a) only occurs in females as a degenerative disorder; (b) is not a disorder.
21. (d) is correct. (a) and (b) are high and low average, respectively; and (c) would be considered low borderline.
22. (a) is correct. (b) is loss of oxygen to the brain; (c) a cognitive developmental disorder; and (d) a metabolic disorder that causes neural degeneration and early death.
23. (d) is correct. (a) involves repeating and making up words that sound similar; (b) is the repetition of words; (c) is not a disorder or symptom.

24. (d) is correct. (a) involves writing deficits; (c) is related to problems in speech; and (b) is not a disorder.
25. (b) is correct. (a), (c), and (d) are not related to integration of neural and sensory information.
26. (a) is correct. (b) involves inability to sit still as well as focus attention; (c) involves both inattentiveness and impulsivity; there is no such disorder as (d).
27. (c) is correct. (a) is eating nonfood items; (b) involves problems in regulation of feeding; and (d) is an eating disorder associated with bingeing and either purging or exercising excessively.
28. (c) is correct. (a) is when a child refuses to talk; (b) is a psychotic disorder; and (d) involves eating nonfood items.

CHAPTER 12
COGNITIVE DISORDERS

CHAPTER AT A GLANCE

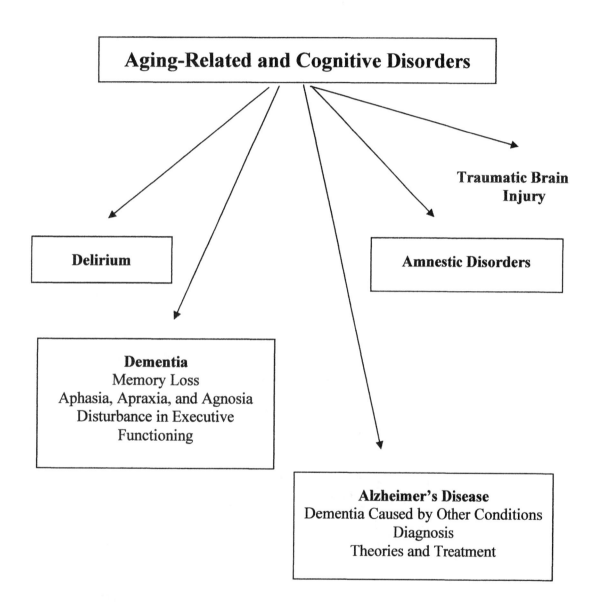

Aging-Related and Cognitive Disorders

Traumatic Brain Injury

Delirium

Amnestic Disorders

Dementia
Memory Loss
Aphasia, Apraxia, and Agnosia
Disturbance in Executive
Functioning

Alzheimer's Disease
Dementia Caused by Other Conditions
Diagnosis
Theories and Treatment

Learning Objectives

1.0   The Nature of Cognitive Disorders
     1.1   Explain the characteristics of disorders involving cognitive impairment.
2.0   Delirium
     2.1   Describe the symptomatic features and possible causes of delirium.
3.0   Amnestic Disorders
     3.1   Outline the types and causes of amnesia.
4.0   Traumatic Brain Injury
     4.1   Indicate some of the causes and characteristics of TBI.
5.0   Dementia
     5.1   Indicate the symptoms of dementia, including memory loss, aphasia, apraxia, agnosia, and disturbance in executive functioning.
6.0   Alzheimer's Disease (Dementia of the Alzheimer's Type)
     6.1   Describe the prevalence, course, and stages of Alzheimer's disease.
     6.2   Indicate other physical diseases and psychological disorders that can lead to dementia resembling Alzheimer's disease.
     6.3   Discuss the issues involved in diagnosing Alzheimer's disease.
     6.4   Contrast the biological and psychological perspectives regarding the causes and treatment of Alzheimer's disease.
7.0   Cognitive Disorders: The Biopsychosocial Perspective
8.0   Chapter Box
     ~~8.1~~   Discuss the case of Iris Murdoch and her husband and caregiver John Bayley.

Identifying the Disorders

Write the name of the cognitive disorder in the blank next to the symptoms listed.

1. _____ Loss of memory for previously learned information or inability to learn new information.

2. _____ Progressive disease of the cortex involving memory loss, aphasia, apraxia, and agnosia.

3. _____ Patchy, stepwise deterioration of intellectual functioning due to cardiovascular disease and reduced blood supply to the brain.

4. _____ Cognitive and personality disturbances accompanied by involuntary spasmodic movements that eventually progress to the point of causing total disability.

5. _____ Symptoms mimicking Alzheimer's disease including depressed mood, disturbances in cognitive functioning, sleep and appetite, anxiety, suicidality, low self-esteem, guilt, and lack of motivation.

6. _____ Temporary disturbance in thoughts, level of consciousness, speech, memory, orientation, perceptions, and motor behavior.

7. _____ Deterioration of parts of the nervous system involved in control of motor movement.

8. _____ Degenerative disease that affects the frontal and temporal lobes of the cortex involving memory loss, social disinhibition, loss of motivation.

9. _____ Recurrent bodily seizures with associated changes in EEG patterns.

10. _____ Rare neurological disease transmitted from animals to humans, leading to dementia

Matching

Put the letter from the right-hand column corresponding to the correct match in the blank next to each item in the left-hand column.

1. ___ Protein that forms the core of plaques found in Alzheimer's.
2. ___ Loss of the ability to carry out coordinated bodily movements.
3. ___ Discoverer of a form of language impairment in which the ability to produce language is lost.
4. ___ Physician who first identified senile dementia.
5. ___ Extreme muscle rigidity involving difficulty in initiating movement.
6. ___ Loss of memories for events prior to brain injury or damage.
7. ___ Neurological condition involving seizures and EEG abnormalities.
8. ___ Substance in the nervous system essential for the formation of acetylcholine.
9. ___ Loss of the ability to use language.
10. ___ Experimental drug used to treat Alzheimer's disease by altering levels of acetylcholine.
11. ___ Inability to recognize familiar objects or events.
12. ___ Discoverer of a form of language impairment in which comprehension abilities is lost.
13. ___ Loss of memories for events taking place after brain damage has occurred.
14. ___ Condition seen in neurons affected by Alzheimer's disease in which tiny strands form in the cell body.
15. ___ Loss or depletion of oxygen to the brain.

a. retrograde amnesia
b. Wernicke
c. epilepsy
d. aphasia
e. neurofibrillary tangles
f. agnosia
g. beta amyloid
h. anoxia
i. anterograde amnesia
j. tacrine (tetrahydro-aminoacrdine)
k. Alzheimer
l. akinesia
m. apraxia
n. Broca
o. choline acetyltransferase

Not-So-Trivial Pursuits Game

This "puzzle" follows the lines of the popular board game in which players must answer questions within a set of six categories. Answer the following questions within these categories.

SL = Sports & Leisure
AL = Arts & Literature
E = Entertainment

H = History
G = Geography
S = Science and Nature

CARD 1:

SL	What disease makes it impossible for people to engage in finely tuned motor activities such as those required for athletics and many hobbies?
AL	What is the name of a book written by Oliver Sacks describing people with various forms of brain damage or other neuropsychological disorders?
E	Who is the former actor who became president and was later diagnosed with Alzheimer's Disease?
H	Which neurologist discovered a form of aphasia in which the individual can produce but not comprehend language?
G	What is the country in which Alzheimer's disease was first discovered?
S	Which neurotransmitter system is thought to be most affected by Alzheimer's disease?

CARD 2:

SL	What is the metal in cooking utensils regarded by some as the basis for Alzheimer's disease?
AL	Who is the author of *The Shattered Mind* which presented lengthy interviews of people with various forms of aphasia?
E	What communication systems are useful for providing support to family members of Alzheimer's patients?
H	What is the year in which Alzheimer's disease was first identified?
G	What group serves as the research sample of 700 nuns whose rate of Alzheimer's disease is lower than in the general population?
S	What part of the brain is thought to be most affected by the degenerative processes associated with Alzheimer's disease?

Short Answer

1. Describe three approaches to diagnosing Alzheimer's disease, including their intended purpose and problems associated with each:

Diagnostic approach	Intended purpose	Problems

2. List the eight major physical diseases or disorders that can mimic Alzheimer's disease, the nature of the disease or disorder involved in each, and how its symptoms differ from Alzheimer's:

Physical disease or disorder	Nature of disease or disorder	How symptoms differ from Alzheimer's disease

3. Summarize the genetic theories for each subtype of Alzheimer's disease, indicating the gene involved and the biochemical effect of the proposed genetic abnormality:

Type of Alzheimer's Disease	Proposed gene	Biochemical effect
Early-onset familial dementia (ages 30 to 60)		
Early-onset familial dementia (ages 40 to 65)		
Late-onset dementia (age 65 plus)		

4. For each of the following forms of treatment or interventions for Alzheimer's disease, describe its goals and methods of implementation:

Treatment or intervention	Goals	Methods of implementation
Community services		
Medications		
Caregiver support		
Behavioral treatment		
Cognitive-behavioral interventions		
Telephone information and referral services; computer networks		

5. How might each of the following indicators be used to differentiate depression (pseudodementia) from dementia due to Alzheimer's disease?

Indicator	Use in differentiating pseudodementia from dementia
Memory complaints	
Order of symptom development	
Nature of symptoms	
Exploration of recent life events	

6. Answer the following questions about the general category of cognitive disorders:

a. How was the term *organic* previously used in the context of psychological disorders?

_____

_____

b. Why did the *DSM-IV* move to the term "delirium, dementia, amnestic, and other cognitive disorders" rather than "organic disorders" to describe disorders caused by brain damage or disease?

_____

_____

c. Provide four examples of psychological symptoms that can be caused by physical abnormalities:

_____   _____

_____   _____

d. What is the primary difficulty involved in diagnosing a cognitive disorder?

_____

_____

e. Why has epilepsy been inaccurately viewed for centuries as a psychological disorder?

_____

_____

7. Contrast delirium with dementia in terms of the following:

	Delirium	Dementia
Cause		
Course		
Primary symptoms		
Outcome		

8. Write in the blank next to the symptom the stage of dementia in which it first becomes evident, using the following symbols:

F   =   Forgetfulness   MD = Middle dementia
EC =   Early confusional   LD = Late dementia
ED =   Early dementia   LC = Late Confusion

Stage	Symptom	Stage	Symptom
_____	Difficulty choosing clothes	_____	Withdrawal from challenging situation
_____	Mild forgetfulness and appropriate concern	_____	Becoming totally dependent on caregiver
_____	Getting lost in familiar places	_____	Complete deterioration of social skills
_____	Forgets name of spouse	_____	Some date and time disorientation
_____	Forgets telephone number	_____	Incapable of self-toileting
_____	Denial of memory problems but with anxiety	_____	Obvious denial of memory problems
_____	Losing ability to handle finances	_____	Loss of all verbal abilities
_____	Occasional but not serious memory lapses	_____	Poor reading comprehension
		_____	Loss of ability to walk
		_____	Family notices forgetfulness

Focusing on Research

Answer the following questions from "What Researchers are Learning from Aging Nuns…"

1. What is idea density, and how is it important?

_____

_____

2. What is meant by "exercising the brain"?

_____

_____

3. What is the role of positive emotional expression?

_____

_____

From the Case Files of Dr. Sarah Tobin: Thinking About Irene's Case

Answer the following questions about the case of Irene Heller.

1. List Irene's symptoms, as observed by Dr. Tobin, during her first meeting and as reported by Jonathan Heller.

   _____

   _____

2. Describe the results of Irene's neuropsychological assessment.

   _____

   _____

3. Discuss the nature and course of the interventions undertaken to help deal with Irene's Alzheimer's disease.

   _____

   _____

Review at a Glance

Test your knowledge by completing the blank spaces with terms from the chapter. If you need a hint, consult the chapter summary.

Cognitive disorders are characterized by (1) _____ that is caused by (2) _____ trauma, (3) _____, or (4) _____.

People with (5) _____ are (6) _____, have (7) _____ memories, and may have various other symptoms such as (8) _____ speech, (9) _____, (10) _____, and (11) _____ disturbances. Delirium is caused by a change in the (12) _____ of the brain and can result from various factors, including (13) _____ or _____, (14) _____ injury, high (15) _____, and (16) _____ deficiency. The onset is (17) _____ and the duration (18) _____.

People with (19) _____ disorders are unable to recall (20) _____ information or register (21) _____. (22) _____ use or medical conditions such as (23) _____ trauma, loss of (24) _____, or (25) _____ cause these disorders.

Dementia involves progressive deficits in a person's (26) _____ and learning of (27) _____, ability to (28) _____, (29) _____, and motor (30) _____. People with dementia also undergo changes in their (31) _____ and (32) _____ state, in addition to cognitive changes. Dementia is the result of profuse and progressive (33) _____ damage, associated with physical conditions such as (34) _____ diseases, (35) _____, (36) _____ trauma, (37) _____ substances, and various (38) _____ disorders. The most well known form of dementia is (39) _____, a condition associated with severe (40) _____ and (41) _____ changes in the brain. The four subtypes of Alzheimer's are: with (42) _____, with (43) _____, with (44) _____ and (45) _____. Theories about the cause of Alzheimer's focus on (46) _____ abnormalities involving the (47) _____ system, specifically changes in the neurons. These are the formation of (48) _____ and the development of (49) _____. Although there is no cure for Alzheimer's disease, medications such as (50) _____ alleviate its symptoms. Psychological interventions involve (51) _____ techniques for managing symptoms and strategies for alleviating (52) _____ burden.

Multiple Choice

1. Which of the following statements is true about people with AIDS who develop dementia?
    a. Education can reduce fear and prejudice against these individuals.
    b. They are likely to encounter accurate knowledge and understanding from society.
    c. Attitudes toward their condition are not related to attitudes toward gays and lesbians.
    d. They receive preferential treatment in housing, employment, and health care.

2. The term *organic* in regard to psychological disorders was traditionally used to refer to
    a. birth defects.
    b. physical illness.
    c. brain damage or dysfunction.
    d. refusal to eat pesticide-treated food.

3. Delirium is caused by
    a. changes in the metabolism of the brain.
    b. intense levels of emotional stress.
    c. too much sleep.
    d. dietary imbalance.

4. Individuals with anterograde amnesia suffer memory loss
    a. due to a traumatic emotional experience.
    b. as a result of epilepsy.
    c. for events prior to their amnesia.
    d. for new events that take place after the amnesia.

5. Controversy regarding chemical restraints for dementia patients centers on
    a. the ethics and wisdom of using medication for restraint.
    b. whether such methods are as effective as physical restraints.
    c. the high cost of these medications when used on a daily basis.
    d. the fact that they are more humane than behavioral treatments.

6. Which symptom is not commonly noted in people with dementia?
    a. aphasia
    b. apraxia
    c. agnosia
    d. anoxia

7. Which of the following statements about Alzheimer's disease is accurate?
    a. The number of cases has decreased.
    b. Women have higher rates of this disorder.
    c. It affects 25 percent of the U.S. population.
    d. The rate is lowest in those over 85.

8. Clusters of dead neurons mixed together with fragments of protein molecules in the brains of people with Alzheimer's disease are called
    a. amyloid plaques.
    b. neurofibrillary tangles.
    c. granulovacuoles.
    d. senillaries.

9. What is the name of the disorder which is a hereditary condition involving a widespread deterioration of the subcortical brain structures and parts of the frontal cortex that control motor movements?
   a. Parkinson's disease
   b. Huntington's disease
   c. Creutzfeldt's syndrome
   d. Brady's kinesia

10. Vascular dementia shows this characteristic pattern?
    a. pseudodementia
    b. patchy deterioration
    c. hydrocephalus
    d. sclerosis

11. Clinicians who provide services to families in which one member has Alzheimer's disease have focused increasingly on:
    a. shared environmental toxins.
    b. genetic predispositions.
    c. the problem of pseudodementia.
    d. caregiver burden.

12. Dependence on caregiver, delusional symptoms, and loss of awareness of all recent events first occur in which stage of dementia?
    a. middle
    b. early
    c. forgetfulness
    d. late

13. Jeremy, a person with epilepsy, has seizures during which he loses consciousness, stops breathing for a short period of time, and experiences body jerking. Jeremy has what type of seizures?
    a. petit mal
    b. generalized convulsive
    c. partial
    d. focal

14. Annie is a 78-year-old woman seen in the Emergency Room who is delusional, is unable to remember her last name, and slurs her speech. Her heart rate is rapid, and she is sweating, but she is not intoxicated. From what might she be suffering?
    a. amnesia
    b. Alzheimer's disease
    c. Huntington's disease
    d. delirium

15. Which of the following is the most common cause of amnestic disorder?
    a. chronic alcohol use
    b. chronic marijuana use
    c. head injury
    d. viral infection

16. Aphasia is defined as the loss of ability to
    a. use language.
    b. recognize familiar objects.
    c. carry out verbal instructions.
    d. learn or remember events.

17. On autopsy, it is determined that a woman's cerebral cortex had degenerated, and there were numerous amyloid plaques in the brain tissue. It is likely that this woman suffered from
    a. Alzheimer's disease.
    b. epilepsy.
    c. pseudodementia.
    d. Tay-Sachs disease.

18. Chronic exposure to the fumes of house paints and petroleum fuels can lead to symptoms that mirror which disease?
    a. Alzheimer's disease
    b. AIDS
    c. Tourette's disease
    d. amnesia

19. A link exists between Alzheimer's disease and which inherited disorder?
    a. Down syndrome
    b. autistic disorder
    c. attention-deficit/hyperactivity disorder
    d. pica

20. Why is it often difficult to diagnose organic disorders?
    a. because the individuals who suffer from these disorders often suffer from somatoform disorders as well
    b. because the individuals suffering from these disorders give false information as to their symptoms
    c. because often the symptoms are not recognized by individuals without training in psychiatry
    d. because many of the symptoms of these disorders are similar to those associated with psychological disorders

21. Tony has seizures during which he loses consciousness and experiences occasional twitching of his eyelids. With which type of seizures does Tony suffer?
   a. generalized convulsive
   b. partial
   c. focal
   d. petit mal

22. A condition in which a person's thoughts, level of consciousness, speech, memory, orientation, perceptions, and motor patterns are very confused, unstable, or otherwise grossly disturbed is called
   a. delirium.
   b. dementia.
   c. amnesia.
   d. tachycardia.

23. Disorders involving a biological loss of memory are called
   a. dissociative disorders.
   b. amnestic disorders.
   c. delirium-related disorders.
   d. neuroses.

24. The form of language impairment, in which the individual is able to produce language but has lost the ability to comprehend so that these verbal productions have no meaning, is referred to as
   a. apraxia.
   b. agnosia.
   c. tachycardia.
   d. Wernicke's aphasia.

25. Which of the following statements about the incidence of Alzheimer's disease in the elderly population is true?
   a. Most elderly people will eventually develop Alzheimer's.
   b. A majority of the elderly develop Alzheimer's disease.
   c. Only a small percentage of the elderly develop Alzheimer's disease.
   d. Alzheimer's disease is much more common in middle-aged individuals.

26. The degenerative course of Alzheimer's disease typically can last up to
   a. 10 months.
   b. 10 years.
   c. 20 years.
   d. 30 years.

27. One biological theory proposes that Alzheimer's disease is the result of disruptions in which neurotransmitter system?
   a. the GABA system
   b. the norepinephrine system
   c. the acetylcholine system
   d. the dopaminergic system

28. Supportive therapy may be useful in helping clients with Alzheimer's disease overcome their
   a. debilitating symptoms.
   b. hallucinations and delusions.
   c. neurological deficits.
   d. concerns over personal loss and mortality.

ANSWERS

IDENTIFYING DISORDERS

1. amnestic disorder
2. dementia
3. vascular dementia
4. Huntington's disease
5. pseudodementia
6. Delirium
7. Parkinson's disease
8. Pick's disease
9. epilepsy
10. Creutzfeld-Jacob disease

MATCHING

1.	g	4.	k	7.	c	10.	j	13.	I
2.	m	5.	l	8.	o	11.	f	14.	e
3.	n	6.	a	9.	d	12.	b	15.	h

NOT SO TRIVIAL PURSUITS

CARD 1:

SL	Parkinson's Disease
AL	*The Man Who Mistook His Wife for a Hat*
E	Ronald Reagan
H	Wernicke
G	Germany
S	Acetylcholine

CARD 2:

SL	Aluminum
AL	Howard Gardner
E	Computer networks
H	1907
G	School Sisters of Notre Dame
S	Hippocampus

SHORT ANSWER

1.

Diagnostic approach	Intended purpose	Problems
CAT and PET scans, MRI	Detect structural brain abnormalities (CAT and MRI) and metabolic defects (PET scans).	Measures not sensitive to brain changes specific to Alzheimer's disease.
Neurological and neuropsychological evaluations involving cognitive tests	Identify patterns of abnormalities indicative of brain damage or cognitive processes of memory and learning.	Can be used to help distinguish between pseudodementia and Alzheimer's disease but are not sensitive enough to Alzheimer's to make reliable diagnosis.
Mental status examination	Assess functional deficits associated with Alzheimer's.	Evidence of deficits in areas assessed by the examination is not sufficient basis for diagnosis.

2.

Physical disease or disorder	Nature of disease or disorder	How symptoms differ from Alzheimer's disease
Substance-induced persisting dementia	Brain damage resulting from exposure to toxins in the environment.	Symptoms are progressive but occur in response to specific environmental agents rather than disease.
Dementia due to head trauma	Brain injury	Similar to Alzheimer's but occurs in a more sudden fashion.
Dementia due to HIV disease	Subtle deterioration in cognitive functioning due to AIDS.	In addition to memory problems, symptoms include movement disturbances, delusions, hallucinations, extreme depression, apathy, and social withdrawal.

Physical disease or disorder	Nature of disease or disorder	How symptoms differ from Alzheimer's disease
Pick's disease	Degenerative disease that affects frontal and temporal lobes of cortex.	Personality alterations precede memory problems.
Parkinson's disease	Neuronal degeneration of basal ganglia; deterioration of diffuse areas of cortex may also occur.	Main features are motor disturbances, including akinesia, brady kinesia, shuffling gait, and loss of fine coordination.
Huntington's disease	Deterioration of subcortical brain structures and parts of frontal cortex that control motor movements; degeneration of corpus callosum.	Main symptoms are involuntary spasmodic and often tortuous movements.
Creutzfeldt-Jakob disease	Neurological disease transmitted from animals to humans that leads to dementia and death.	Initial symptoms are fatigue, anxiety, appetite disturbance, sleep problems, and concentration difficulties; disease progression results in loss of motor coordination, vision problems, and further neural disturbance.
Vascular dementia	Death of selected groups of neurons in cerebral cortex when clusters of capillaries in the brain are cut off by infarctions.	Patchy, stepwise cognitive deterioration.

3.

Type of Alzheimer's disease	Proposed gene	Biochemical effect
Early-onset familial dementia (ages 30 to 60)	Presenilin genes (PS1 on chromosome 14 and PS 2 on chromosome 1)	Codes a protein embedded in a membrane of the neuron that might be involved in protein transport between neurons and possibly connected with amyloid plaques.
Early-onset familial dementia (ages 40 to 65)	APP gene on chromosome 21	Interference with disposal mechanism for APP might lead to accumulation of beta-amyloid protein and eventual formation of amyloid plaques.
Late-onset dementia (age 65 plus)	APOE on chromosome 19	The APo E 4 allele codes for the E4 form of Apo E which may damage the microtubles within the neuron that play an essential role in transport throughout the cell; this damage may occur through the destruction of the tau protein which stabilizes the microtubules.

4.

Treatment or intervention	Goals	Methods of implementation
Community services	Maintain the individual for as long as possible at current level of functioning	Diagnostic and medical assessment, counseling, support groups, financial planning assistance, and home care services; day care and respite programs to aid caregivers
Medications	Offset the effects of the disease on the brain	Vasodilators or metabolic enhancers to increase blood flow to the brain, choline-based substances to increase activity of acetylcholine; tacrine, which decreases the activity of cholinesterase
Caregiver support	Help caregivers work through feelings of guilt and anger and other intense emotional reactions	Insight-oriented psychotherapy
Behavioral treatment	Maximize individual's ability to adapt to the environment and maintain independence	Teach daily living skills (dressing, bathing, cooking, and social skills) and reduce disruptive behaviors (wandering and incontinence)
Cognitive-behavioral interventions	Alleviate depression in afflicted individual and caregivers	Focus on compensation for memory problems and help caregivers with feelings of depression caused by dysfunctional attitudes about their role in treating the individual
Telephone information and referral services; computer networks	Provide caregivers with information as well as emotional support	Informal sharing of help and information in a readily accessible format

5.

Indicator	Use in differentiating pseudodementia from dementia
Memory complaints	Depressed individuals complain about their faulty memory, even though there is no physical basis for their complaints; the individual with Alzheimer's tries to conceal or minimize the extent of impairment or explain it away. As the disease progresses, the Alzheimer's patient may even falsely sense an improvement of memory functioning.
Order of symptom development	In depressed elderly people, mood changes precede memory loss; the reverse is true for Alzheimer's patients.
Nature of symptoms	People with pseudodementia show classic symptoms of depression, including anxiety, sleep and appetite disturbance, suicidal thoughts, low self-esteem, guilt, and lack of motivation. Their memory problems come on suddenly, and they may have a history of depression. People with dementia experience unsociability, uncooperative-ness, hostility, emotional instability, confusion, disorientation, and reduced alertness. The course of memory impairment is gradual and progressive.
Exploration of recent life events	Depressed elderly persons are more likely to have suffered a recent stressful life event; life events are not thought to be a factor in the development of dementia.

6.
a. The term *organic* was traditionally used in psychology to refer to physical damage or dysfunction that affects the integrity of the brain.
b. Movement away from the term *organic* was suggested in recognition of the fact that many psychological disorders have their origins in brain dysfunction. The current term more accurately describes the nature of the dysfunction in this group of disorders.
c. hallucinations
   delusions
   mood disturbances
   extreme personality changes
d. It is difficult to differentiate symptoms associated with a psychological disorder from those arising in response to a physical disorder even with the aid of sophisticated diagnostic technology.
e. Epilepsy has been misunderstood as a psychological disorder because people with this disorder may act in ways that appear odd or psychotic.

7.

	Delirium	Dementia
Cause	Change in metabolism of the brain.	Progressive degeneration of the cortex
Course	Rapid onset and brief duration.	Slow onset and long duration
Primary symptoms	Any or all of the following psychological changes: confusion, disturbance of consciousness, delusions, illusions, hallucinations, and emotional disturbances as well as autonomic nervous system disturbance.	Loss of memory, language abilities, orientation, motor abilities, judgment, and social skills as well as emotional instability.
Outcome	Positive outcomes are possible such as natural recovery or positive response to treatment unless the delirium reflects a neurological disease or life-threatening condition	Death invariably occurs due to the development of secondary physical illness.

8.

ED	MD	LC	MD	LD	EC
F	ED	F	LD	LC	LD
EC	EC	LC	ED	LD	EC

FOCUSING ON RESEARCH

1. Idea density is the number of ideas per given number of written words. It proved to be a powerful predictor of which nuns would develop Alzheimer's disease.
2. The brain can be exercised by performing frequent cognitive activity. Nuns who were cognitively active as teachers showed less cognitive decline than those who performed less cognitively active duties.
3. Those nuns who often expressed positive emotions such as love, hope, gratitude, and contentment tended to live longer than did those who expressed more negative emotions.

FROM THE CASE FILES OF DR. SARAH TOBIN: THINKING ABOUT IRENE'S CASE

1. Memory problems, anger, confusion, paranoia, and denial that she had any problem other than being a little "forgetful."
2. Moderate cognitive deficits, problems with abstract reasoning and verbal fluency, disorientation as to time and place, memory impairment, and depression.

3.   The diagnosis was Dementia of the Alzheimer's type. The treatment plan involved moving into an assisted-living apartment complex; multidisciplinary assistance from a psychologist, social worker, and counselor from the local Counsel of Aging; and assistance with self-care and independent living. She deteriorated rapidly and progressively. After 6 months in the assisted-living residence, she was moved to a nursing home because she was a danger to herself and others. She deteriorated to the point that she rarely recognized her son.

REVIEW AT A GLANCE

1. cognitive impairment
2. brain disease
4. exposure to toxic substances
5. delirium
6. disoriented
7. foggy
8. rambling
9. delusions
10. hallucinations
11. emotional
12. metabolism
13. intoxication; withdrawal
14. head
15. fever
16. vitamin
17. rapid
18. brief

19. amnestic
20. previously learned
21. new memories
22. substance
23. head
24. oxygen
25. herpes simplex
26. memory
27. new information
28. communicate
29. judgment
30. coordination
31. personality
32. emotional
33. brain
34. vascular
35. AIDS

36. head
37. psychoactive
38. neurological
39. Alzheimer's disease
40. cerebral atrophy
41. microscopic
42. delirium
43. delusions
44. depressed mood
45. uncomplicated
46. biological
47. nervous
48. neurofibrillary tangles
49. amyloid plaques
50. anticholinesterase
51. behavioral
52. caregiver

MULTIPLE CHOICE

1.   (a) is correct. (b), (c), and (d) are not true.
2.   (c) is correct. (a), (b), and (d) are unrelated to the term.
3.   (a) is correct. (b), (c), and (d) are not known causes of delirium.
4.   (d) is correct. (a), (b), and (c) refer to other types of amnesia.
5.   (a) is correct. There is no controversy concerning (b); (c) and (d) are not accurate statements.
6.   (d) is correct. (a), (b), and (c) may be associated with dementia, but (d) is loss of oxygen to the brain.
7.   (a) is correct. (b), (c), and (d) are not accurate statements.
8.   (a) is correct. (b) and (c) refer to other neurological states; there is no such thing as (d).
9.   (a) is correct. (b), (c), and (d) are not associated with the described symptoms.
10. (b) is correct. (a) refers to false dementia; (c) to water on the brain; and (d) to a degenerative motor condition.
11. (d) is correct. (a), (b), and (c) are etiological and diagnostic issues, but only (d) is related to services to families.
12. (a) is correct. (c) is not a stage because the individuals suffering from these disorders give false information as to their symptoms ; there is little dependence in (b) and there is total deterioration in (d).
13. (b) is correct. (a), (c), and (d) may have some, but not all, of the described occurrences.
14. (d) is correct. (a), (b), and (c) would not be indicated by these symptoms.
15. (a) is correct. (b), (c), and (d) may cause memory loss, but not to the degree that (a) does.16 (a) is correct. (b) refers to agnosia; (c) to apraxia; and (d) to amnesia.
16. (a) is correct. (b), (c), and (d) would not be associated with this neurological symptom
17. (a) is correct. (b), (c), and (d) are not related to this environmental condition.
18. (a) is correct. (b), (c), and (d) are not associated with the described symptom.
19. (a) is correct. (b), (c), and (d) are not related to Alzheimer's disease.
20. (d) is correct. There is no support for (a), (b), and (c).
21. (d) is correct. (a), (b), and (c) do not involve the exact conditions described
22. (a) is correct. (b) and (c) both involve memory impairment; (d) involves a heart-related disorder.
23. (b) is correct. (a), (c), and (d) are not related to memory loss.

24. (d) is correct. (a) involves inability to form purposeful bodily actions; (b) is the failure to recognize things; and (c) is a heart-related condition.
25. (c) is correct. There is no support for (a), (b), and (d).
26. (b) is correct. (a) is an underestimate; (c) and (d) overestimates.
27. (c) is correct. Alzheimer's has not been related to (a), (b), or (d).
28. (d) is correct. Supportive therapy cannot benefit (a), (b), and (c).

Identifying the Substance

Write the name of the substance that is described in the right-hand column.

1. _____ A stimulant drug that was an ingredient of a popular soft drink during the late 1800s.
2. _____ The most widely used illegal drug in the United States.
3. _____ An opioid whose use had declined steadily from a peak in the 1970s but which appears to be on the rise again.
4. _____ Even if used appropriately as anesthetics, anticonvulsants, and sleeping pills, drugs in this category have high addictive potential.
5. _____ 10% of adults in the United States abuse or are dependent on this substance.
6. _____ A stimulant ingested daily by at least 85% of the U.S. adult population.
7. _____ Hallucinogen that was a central component of the nationwide drug culture of the 1960s.
8. _____ An inexpensive form of a stimulant drug whose use skyrocketed in the 1980s due to its availability on the streets and inaccurate perception of its risk.
9. _____ The yearly cost of abuse of this substance in the U.S. averages at least $100 billion.
10. _____ A category of stimulant drugs whose legitimate medical use is appetite suppression, control of hyperactivity in children, and control of narcolepsy.

Matching

Put the letter from the right-hand column corresponding to the correct match in the blank next to each item in the left-hand column.

1. ___ Physiological and psychological reactions that can occur when a psychoactive substance is discontinued.
2. ___ Proposed subcategory of alcohol dependence theorized to be caused almost exclusively by genetic factors.
3. ___ The extent to which an individual requires larger doses of a substance to achieve its desired effects.
4. ___ A program that provides support and understanding for relatives and friends of people with alcohol dependence.
5. ___ Physiological factor that influences the extent to which a given amount of alcohol will have psychoactive effects.
6. ___ A psychological and physical need for a psychoactive substance.
7. ___ Alteration in behavior due to the accumulation of a psychoactive substance in the body.
8. ___ A pattern of drug use that creates significant problems for a person in everyday life.
9. ___ Physical condition involving autonomic system dysfunction, confusion, and seizures caused by withdrawal from long-term heavy use of alcohol.

a. methaqualone
b. dependence
c. membrane hypothesis
d. Type 1 alcoholism
e. ACOA
f. intoxication
g. expectancy model
h. delirium tremens
i. tolerance
j. Al-Anon
k. substance abuse
l. metabolism rate
m. Type 2 alcoholism
n. withdrawal
o. abstinence violation effect

10. ___ Proposed subcategory of alcohol dependence caused by a hereditary predisposition interacting with environmental causes.

11. ___ Explanation of the biological mechanisms of alcohol that focuses on the changes in the body's cells caused by intake of alcohol.

12. ___ Psychological explanation of alcohol use proposing that a combination of beliefs about the effects of alcohol and reinforcement for these beliefs leads to alcohol dependence.

13. ___ Social movement that raised awareness of the impact of alcoholism on family members (abbreviation).

14. ___ The interpretation of a lapse by an alcohol dependent individual as a lack of ability to control drinking.

15. ___ Non-barbiturate substance with high abuse potential originally designed to replace barbiturates.

Diamond Puzzle

The clues below are all for the "across" direction this puzzle. Clue #1 is for the first row, #2 for the second row, and so on.

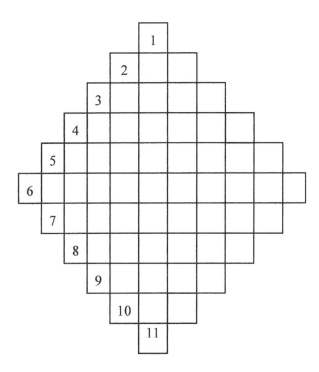

1. First letter of the abbreviation for a treatment approach for alcohol dependence which emphasizes commitment to group meetings, support networks, and spirituality.
2. Abbreviation for one of two enzymes that is responsible for metabolizing alcohol.
3. Use of a psychoactive substance in a way that places the individual at significant risk or harm in daily life.
4. Residential treatment program founded in the late 1950s based on the principle that substance dependent individuals benefit from a therapeutic community approach.
5. A drug that has THC as its active ingredient.
6. A drug used in treating alcohol dependence that is intended to reduce the desire for alcohol by acting on the GABA system.
7. Extent to which the individual can ingest larger amounts of a psychoactive substance without feeling its effects.
8. Stimulant drug thought to cause a "high" by blocking the reuptake in the nervous system of excitatory neurotransmitters, leading to stimulation of pleasure reward centers in the brain.
9. When the effects of cocaine wear off, a person is likely to experience a _____.
10. Hallucinogenic drug accidentally discovered by a scientist that became a central part of the 1960s drug culture.
11. Second letter of the abbreviation for the treatment approach for alcohol dependence in item 1.

Short Answer

1. List six types of medications used in the treatment of alcohol dependence and the intended effect of each medication.

Medication	Intent

2. For each of the following psychoactive substances, describe: (a) its subjective effects, (b) whether it has potential for tolerance and dependence, (c) whether there are withdrawal effects when it is discontinued, and (d) risks or long-term effects (apart from the dangers associated with withdrawal):

Psychoactive Substance	Subjective Effects	Tolerance and Dependence	Withdrawal	Risks or long-term effects
Alcohol		Yes/No	Yes/No	
Amphetamines		Yes/No	Yes/No	
Cocaine		Yes/No	Yes/No	
Cannabis (Marijuana)		Yes/No	Yes/No	
Hallucinogens		Yes/No	Yes/No	
Opioids		Yes/No	Yes/No	
Barbiturates		Yes/No	Yes/No	
Barbiturate-like substances		Yes/No	Not discussed	
Anxiolylitics		Yes/No	Yes/No	

3. Link the terms in the left-hand column with the terms on the right by drawing a line from the term on the left to the matching term on the right. Explain how they are related to each other on the line that matches the term on the left:

How Terms Are Related

Wernicke	Caffeine
Cue Exposure	Enkephalins
Cocaine	Withdrawal
Endorphins	Korsakoff
Tolerance	Relapse Prevention

4. Discuss the kinds of risks or accidents that result from the abuse of alcohol (be as specific as you can).

   _____

   _____

   _____

5. Summarize the evidence for a biological theory of alcohol dependence in terms of each of the following areas of investigation:

Area of Investigation	Available evidence
Patterns of Inheritance	
Biological Matters	
Neurotransmitter Functioning	
Search for an "alcohol" gene	

6. What are four obstacles that stand in the way of recovery for substance abusers?

   _____

   _____

7. a. What is the central assumption of the relapse prevention model?

   _____

   _____

   c. Four areas of focus involved in the relapse prevention model for treating alcohol dependence are:

   _____

   _____

   d. What are the two central assumptions of Alcoholics Anonymous?

   _____

   _____

   e. What four areas of treatment are similar in both the relapse prevention model and Alcoholics Anonymous?

   _____

   _____

f. In what two approaches to treatment does relapse prevention differ from Alcoholics Anonymous?

Alcholics Anonymous	Relapse Prevention

Focusing on Research

Answer the following questions from "Research Focus: How Dangerous is Ecstasy?"

1. What effects of MDMA make it appealing to users?

_____

_____

2. What are some of the medical risks of MDMA use?

_____

_____

3. What are some of the psychological effects on heavy users of MDMA?

_____

_____

From the Case Files of Dr. Sarah Tobin: Thinking About Carl's Case

Answer the following questions about the case of Carl Wadsworth.

1. How was cocaine use negatively impacting Carl's life?

_____

_____

2. What was Dr. Tobin's formulation of Carl's case?

_____

_____

3. Discuss the course and outcome of Carl's treatment.

_____

_____

Social Context

Answer the following questions from the text box, "The Influence of Race and Culture on Alcoholism."

1. Identify the general different patterns of drinking in European and American societies.

    _____

    _____

2. What might help explain the comparative differences in alcohol-related problems of African American and Caucasian men?

    _____

    _____

3. What are two reasons that help account for lower rates of alcoholism in some Asian countries relative to Western nations?

    _____

    _____

4. How do patterns of alcohol use differ for men and women, generally speaking?

    _____

    _____

Review at a Glance

Test your knowledge by completing the blank spaces with terms from the chapter. If you need a hint, consult the chapter summary.

A substance is a chemical that alters a person's (1) _____ or (2) _____ when (3) _____, (4) _____, (5) _____, (6) _____, or (7) _____. Substance (8) _____ is a temporary experience of (9) _____ or (10) _____ changes due to the accumulation of the substance in the body. When some substances are discontinued, some people may experience symptoms of substance (11) _____ that involve (12) _____ and (13) _____ changes. Individuals who experience these changes may develop a (14) _____ for the substance. Substance (15) _____ is the maladaptive pattern of use that leads to significant (16) _____ or (17) _____.

The short-term effect of alcohol is appealing because of its (18) qualities. Long-term use can cause serious harm to many (19) _____ of the body and can lead to (20) _____ problems and (21) _____. Researchers in the field of alcohol dependence first proposed the (22) _____ model of psychological disorder. The biological factor is most likely (23) _____. Psychological theories about alcohol dependence focus concepts derived from (24)

_____, (25) _____, (26) _____ perspectives. According to the (27) _____ model, people develop problematic beliefs about alcohol early in life through (28) _____ and (29) _____ learning. The sociocultural perspective emphasizes the stressors within the (30) _____, (31) _____, and (32) _____ as factors that lead to alcohol dependence.

      Biological treatments for alcohol problems include mediations to control (33) _____ symptoms and (34) _____ agents that provoke nausea after alcohol ingestion. Psychological interventions focus on (35) _____ and (36) _____ techniques. (37)_____ is a (38) _____ program built on the premise that alcohol is a (39) _____.

      (40)_____ have an (41) _____ effect on the nervous system. (42)_____ in moderate amounts cause feelings of (43) _____, increased (44) _____, (45) _____ and (46) _____. In moderate doses, (47) _____ leads to feelings of (48) _____, (49) _____ excitement, (50) _____, (51) _____, and (52) _____. (53)_____ symptoms can develop with higher use of stimulants and cocaine. (54)_____ or marijuana, causes altered (55)_____, and (56)_____ sensations, as well as maladaptive (57) _____ and (58) _____ reactions. (59) _____ cause abnormal (60) _____ experiences in the form of (61) _____ and (62) _____. (63) _____ users experience intense (64) _____ sensations. (65) _____, (66) _____, (67) _____ induce relaxation, sleep, tranquility, and reduced awareness.

      Biological treatment for substance-related disorders involve (68) _____ that block or reduce (69) _____. Behavioral treatments involve techniques such as (70) _____, while cognitive-behavioral techniques are used to help clients modify their (71) _____, (72) _____, and (73) _____ associated with drug use.

Multiple Choice

1. Jared has found that he needs to drink 4 or 5 beers to achieve the level of relaxation that he was able to achieve with only two beers a year ago. This phenomenon is called
   a. withdrawal.
   b. intoxication.
   c. potentiation.
   d. tolerance.

2. Which of the following is not associated with the rate at which alcohol is absorbed into the bloodstream?
   a. concentration of alcohol in a beverage
   b. time of day when alcohol is consumed
   c. metabolic rate of the individual
   d. mixing a carbonated beverage with alcohol

3. Which of the following has contributed to the hypothesis of a genetic link in the development of alcoholism?
   a. Sons of alcoholics are four times more likely to become alcoholic than sons of nonalcoholics.
   b. Daughters of alcoholics are three times more likely to become alcoholic than daughters of nonalcoholics.
   c. Fraternal twins have a higher concordance rate for alcoholism than identical twins.
   d. Children of alcoholics have a stronger reaction to alcohol than children of nonalcoholics.

4. Marianne takes a medication that gives her a headache, nausea, and other unpleasant symptoms each time she has alcohol. This medication is
   a. disulfiram.
   b. nalxetrone.
   c. acamprosate.
   d. aldehyde.

5. Compared to amphetamines, the stimulating effects of cocaine are
   a. longer but less intense.
   b. shorter but more intense.
   c. longer but more intense.
   d. similar in duration and intensity.

6. This term describes the experience in which a cocaine user develops convulsions because the brain's threshold for seizures has been lowered by repeated exposure.
   a. tolerance
   b. intoxication
   c. kindling
   d. potentiation

7. Cross-cultural research on patterns of alcohol use and abuse has shown that:
   a. rates of alcohol abuse are remarkably stable across cultures.
   b. Asian societies discourage alcohol use among men.
   c. prevalence rates are highest among the Amish in America.
   d. cultural and social deprivations can contribute to high rates of abuse.

8. Opioids are also known as:
   a. narcotics.
   b. hallucinogens.
   c. sedatives
   d. hypnotics.

9. The most frequently used drug in the category of barbiturate-like substances is
   a. clonazepam.
   b. secobarbital.
   c. diazepam.
   d. methaqualone.

10. Which of the following statements is true regarding research on babies whose mothers used crack cocaine when pregnant?
    a. It is difficult to separate the effects of crack from those of other substances.
    b. These infants have higher birth weight and larger head size.
    c. Early intervention cannot alter the developmental course of a crack baby's life.
    d. Withdrawal effects are shown in the infants for at least the first year of life.

11. What is the term used for programs that are intended to minimize the physiological changes associated with withdrawal from substances?
    a. milieu
    b. therapeutic community
    c. Alcoholics Anonymous
    d. detoxification

12. Psychologists who have tried to validate the existence of an "addictive personality" have found that
    a. this construct cannot be clearly identified.
    b. such individuals are unlikely to be depressed.
    c. such individuals are addicted to substances but not food.
    d. an individual's personality is linked to physiological factors.

13. The physical and psychological changes that accompany discontinuation of a psychoactive substance are referred to as:
    a. tolerance.
    b. intoxication.
    c. withdrawal.
    d. potentiation.

14. When two or more psychoactive substances are combined, the intoxicant effect can be greater than the effect due to each substance acting alone, a situation referred to as:
    a. sedation.
    b. inebriation.
    c. metabolism.
    d. potentiation.

15. Paul is a chronic alcoholic with dementia. He also has difficulties remembering past events and forming new memories. He suffers from:
    a. Type 1 Alcoholism.
    b. Alzheimer's disease.
    c. Wernicke's disease.
    d. Korsakoff's syndrome.

16. Joyce is alcohol dependent and trying to abstain from drinking. However, she went to a party, broke down, and had a drink. According to the expectancy model, how should she view this behavior?
    a. She should view it as a sign of a character flaw.
    b. She should view it as a sign of personal weakness.
    c. She should not view it as a result of social pressure.
    d. She should not view it as a loss of self-control.

17. Which treatment program is heavily grounded in spirituality?
    a. Alcoholics Anonymous
    b. cue exposure method
    c. relapse prevention therapy
    d. detoxification

18. Amphetamines enhance the action of which neurotransmitter?
    a. serotonin
    b. norepinephrine
    c. GABA
    d. dopamine

19. Spontaneous hallucinations, delusions, or disturbances in mood that are not the result of ingestion of a hallucinogen are called:
    a. psychotic breaks.
    b. delirium tremens.
    c. flashbacks.
    d. illusory spasms.

20. Enkephalins and endorphins are:
    a. natural pain-killing substances produced by the brain.
    b. narcotics.
    c. hallucinogens.
    d. produced only in heavy narcotic users.

21. The experience of altered behaviors due to the accumulation of a substance in the body is referred to as
    a. tolerance.
    b. intoxication.
    c. withdrawal.
    d. dependence.

22. Which of the following is the main feature of substance abuse?
    a. use of a substance in order to prevent withdrawal
    b. continued use of a drug despite risks or problems in living
    c. usage of increased amounts of a drug to achieve the same high
    d. subjective feeling of a need for the substance

23. Dwayne went out drinking despite the fact that he has been taking sleeping pills. As a consequence, he has lapsed into a coma. Dwayne has experienced the effects of drug
    a. abuse.
    b. dependence.
    c. tolerance.
    d. potentiation.

24. The permanent form of dementia in which the individual develops retrograde and anterograde amnesia, leading to an inability to remember recent events or learn new information is called:
    a. Wernicke's disease.
    b. Broca's disease.
    c. Korsakoff's syndrome.
    d. Tourette's syndrome.

25. Which neurotransmitter system may be involved in the effects of alcohol?
    a. the norepinephrine system
    b. the GABA system
    c. the enkephalin system
    d. the cholinergic system

26. According to Woititz, which one of the following is one of the characteristic behavior patterns apparent in adult children of alcoholics?
    a. They fail to establish intimate relationships.
    b. They act in extremely antisocial ways.
    c. They are often overly shy and reticent.
    d. They tend to be abusive to their own children.

27. Aldehyde dehydrogenase (ALDH) is
    a. a medication prescribed to treat alcoholism.
    b. the same thing as disulfiram.
    c. an enzyme responsible for the metabolism of alcohol.
    d. a medication used to treat heroin addicts.

28. The condition that develops from chronic abuse of amphetamine, or from one very large doses of amphetamine, is referred to as
    a. schizophrenia.
    b. delirium tremens.
    c. Korsakoff's syndrome.
    d. stimulant psychosis.

29. The most widely abused illegal drug in the United States is
    a. cocaine.
    b. marijuana.
    c. alcohol.
    d. caffeine.

30. The synthetic opioid that produces a safer and more controlled reaction than heroin is referred to as
    a. endorphin.
    b. enkaphalin.
    c. morphine.
    d. methadone.

Answers

IDENTIFYING THE SUBSTANCE

1. cocaine
2. marijuana
3. heroin
4. barbiturates
5. alcohol
6. caffeine
7. LSD
8. crack cocaine
9. alcohol
10. amphetamine

MATCHING

1. n
2. m
3. i.
4. j
5. l
6. b
7. f
8. k
9. h
10. d
11. c
12. g
13. e
14. o
15. a

PUZZLE

```
         A
        A D H
      A B U S E
    S Y N A N O N
  M A R I J U A N A
A C A M P R O S A T E
  T O L E R A N C E
    C O C A I N E
      C R A S H
        L S D
         A
```

SHORT ANSWER

1.

Medication	Intent
Benzodiazepines	Manage symptoms of withdrawal and delirium..
Acamprosate	Reduce desire for alcohol by acting on the GABA neurotransmitter system.
Citalopram	Reduce desire for alcohol by inhibiting the uptake of serotonin.
Buspirone	Reduce desire for alcohol by inhibiting the uptake of serotonin.
Naltrexone	Reduces pleasurable feelings associated with alcohol use by altering opioid receptors.
Disulfiram	Produces aversive reaction to alcohol by causing a violently unpleasant reaction when mixed with alcohol.

2.

Psychoactive Substance	Subjective effects	Tolerance and Dependence	Withdrawal	Risks or long-term effects
Alcohol	**Small amounts**: sedative effects **Larger amounts**: disinhibition **Very large amounts**: sleepiness, uncoordination, dysphoria, irritability	Yes	Yes	Brain damage, liver disease, damage to the gastrointestinal system, osteoporosis, cancer, reduced functioning of immune system.
Amphetamines	**Moderate amounts**: euphoria, confidence, talkativeness, energy. **Large amounts**: surge or "rush" of extremely pleasurable sensations.	Yes	Yes	Amphetamine-induced psychosis, also called stimulant psychosis.
Cocaine	**Moderate doses**: Euphoria, sexual excitement, potency, energy, and talkativeness; **Higher doses**: delusions, hallucinations, confusion, suspicion, agitation, and violence.	Yes	Yes	Heart failure and convulsions.
Cannabis (Marijuana)	**Moderate doses**: relaxation and feeling that time is slowed down, heightened sensual enjoyment, hunger, greater awareness of surroundings, possible impairment of short-term memory; **Higher doses**: visual hallucinations and paranoid delusions.	Not clear from available evidence	No	Nasal and respiratory problems, higher risk of cancer and cardiovascular disease, negative effects on reproductive functioning particularly in men; possible loss of motivation; increased risk of accidents.
Hallucinogens	**LSD**: Dizziness, weakness, euphoria, hallucinations; **Psilocybin**: relaxation and euphoria; **PCP**: low doses like depressant; larger doses cause distorted perceptions that can lead to violence.			**LSD**: Flashbacks and hallucinogen persisting perception disorder. **PCP**: coma, convulsions, brain damage, disorientation so severe that it can lead to accidental death.
Opioids	Intensely pleasurable physical sensations and subjective feelings of euphoria.	Yes	Yes	Highly addictive. Long-term effects: decrease in respiratory efficiency, high blood pressure, and difficulty withdrawing.

Psychoactive Substance	Subjective effects	Tolerance and Dependence	Withdrawal	Risks or long-term effects
Barbiturates	**Low doses**: feeling of calm and sedation, sociability, talkativeness, euphoria. **Higher doses**: sleep.	Yes	Yes	Accidental suicide due to respiratory failure. Alcohol potentiates the effect of these drugs, so risk is greater when they are combined with alcohol.
Barbiturate-like substances	Dissociation, loss of inhibitions, greater euphoria during sexual encounters.	Yes	Not discussed in text	Not discussed in text
Anxiolytics	Calm and relaxation.	Yes	Yes	Text discussion includes only withdrawal symptoms which can be severe.

3. Wernicke and Korsakoff: names of dementias associated with long-term heavy alcohol consumption.
   Cue exposure and relapse prevention: two psychological treatments for alcohol dependence.
   Cocaine and caffeine: stimulants.
   Endorphins and enkephalins: two natural pain-reducing substances in the nervous system.
   Tolerance and withdrawal: two patterns associated with substance dependence.

4. Alcohol is responsible for more than half of the fatal automobile accidents in the U.S.
   Intoxicated pedestrians are four times more likely than nonintoxicated pedestrians to be hit by a car.
   Alcohol increases the risks of accidental drownings, falls, fires, and burns.
   Greater likelihood of serious trauma when an intoxicated person is involved in an accident.
   Increased risk of domestic violence as indicated by the finding that almost two-thirds of husbands who abused their wives were under the influence of alcohol when violent.

5.

Area of investigation	Available evidence
Patterns of inheritance	Higher concordance rate among identical than fraternal twins. Sons of alcoholics are four times more likely to become alcohol dependent than are sons of nonalcoholic parents, and the risk is higher for children of alcoholics regardless of whether they are raised by their biological parents or not.
Biological markers	Subjective reaction to alcohol: Nonalcoholic children of alcoholics show less of a subjective reaction than do children of nonalcoholics. P300 wave: Similar to alcoholics, children of alcoholic fathers show a lowering of the P300 wave after presentation of a stimulus.
Neurotransmitter functioning	Abnormalities have been examined in the GABA, serotonin, and dopamine neurotransmitter systems.
Search for an "alcohol" gene	Attempts have been made to find an "alcohol" gene that influences dopamine receptors but so far, have been unsuccessful.

6. In the case of alcohol dependence, alcohol is so much a part of Western society that people may not even realize that excessive consumption is a problem.
   Alcohol-dependent individuals tend to deny that they have a problem.
   The individual may be unwilling to reveal the problem to others.
   There is an inherently reinforcing property of psychoactive substance use.
   The painful nature of withdrawal symptoms makes it difficult for the user to achieve abstinence.

7.

a. Alcohol-dependent individuals are faced with the temptation to have a drink and at some point fail to abstain; according to the abstinence violation effect, if the individual's self-efficacy is lowered, a relapse is likely.

b. Decision-making for analyzing situations presenting a high risk of alcohol use.
Skills training to express and receive feelings, initiate contact with others, and reply to criticism.
Alternate coping methods for handling high-risk situations.
Self-efficacy for maintaining abstinence.

c. Alcoholism is an illness or disease.
A person never completely recovers from alcoholism, no matter how long abstinence has been maintained.

d. Avoid self-blame for lapses from abstinence.
Develop alternate coping skills for handling situations involving potential alcohol use.
Receive help through support and contact with others.
Be motivated to participate in treatment.

e.

Alcoholics Anonymous	Relapse prevention
Control over drinking is seen as due to an outside force.	Control over drinking is seen as due to internal factors.
The client is encouraged to seek help from outside.	The client learns to draw on personal coping resources.

FOCUSING ON RESEARCH

1. Users report feeling physically and psychologically warm. There is a mellow glow and increased energy.
2. Because body temperature rises with MDMA, users in hot, crowded places risk hyperthermia and even convulsions. There is serotonin depletion, which can alter mood, sleep, pain, and appetite. Imaging studies have shown brain changes such as reduced cerebral blood flow.
3. Users have been found to have long lasting impairments in memory. Heavy users often experience anxiety, aggression, impulsivity, and depression. Longitudinal research is under way to see how many of the changes might be lifelong.

FROM THE CASE FILES OF DR. SARAH TOBIN: THINKING ABOUT CARL'S CASE

1. Financial problems caused by his expensive cocaine habit, spending more time away from home, becoming sloppy in his work as a resident, abrupt and insensitive to patients and nursing staff, losing control of his interactions with his wife and daughter, being irritable and impatient.
2. Carl grew up with intense pressure to become a doctor, as if to be anything else would result in his father's rejection of him. Carl depended on others heavily to succeed, and probably married his wife because he needed a caretaker. She could not help him in his search for greater self-esteem. Carl turned to cocaine, a substance that deluded him into believing that he was happy, competent, and successful.
3. After a four-week in-patient program, he began intensive psychotherapy that was confrontational and cognitive in approach. He was involved in a support group of local physicians with similar problems. He gained insight into his problems, changed his priorities, and made a dramatic improvement.

SOCIAL CONTEXT

1. In some American societies, alcohol use is discouraged or prohibited such as in certain conservative religions and among the Amish. In many European societies, alcohol is integrated into the daily diet and often a standard accompaniment to meals.
2. One study found that African American men and Caucasian men develop alcoholism at similar rates, yet African American men have more alcohol-related problems, including health and interpersonal problems. Disadvantages in health care, employment, and education may contribute to higher alcohol-related problems in African American men.
3. Although some Asian men drink heavily in certain work settings, drinking outside of social situations is often discouraged and women are discouraged from drinking. Further, some members of Asian cultures seem vulnerable to the buildup of potentially toxic by-products of alcohol, making intoxication an unpleasant physical

experience.

4. While men may drink to suppress painful emotions, women seem more likely to drink to escape painful interpersonal situations. In traditional male-dominated societies, such as Hispanic and Asian cultures, there are strong prohibitions against women becoming intoxicated.

REVIEW AT A GLANCE

1. mood	21. dementia	38. 12 step	58. psychological
2. behavior	22. biopsychosocial	39. disease	59. hallucinogens
3. smoked	23. genetic	40. Stimulants	60. perceptual
4. injected	24. behavioral	41. activating	61. illusions
5. drunk	25. cognitive-behavioral	42. Amphetamines	62. hallucinations
6. inhaled		43. euphoria	63. opioid
7. swallowed	26. social learning	44. confidence	64. bodily
8. intoxication	27. expectancy	45. talkativeness	65. sedatives
9. behavioral	28. reinforcement	46. energy	66. hypnotics
10. psychological	29. observational	47. cocaine	67. anxiolytics
11. withdrawal	30. family	48. euphoria	68. medications
12. physical	31. community	49. sexual	69. craving
13. psychological	32. culture	50. potency	70. contingency management
14. tolerance	33. withdrawal	51. energy	
15. abuse	34. aversive	52. talkativeness	71. thoughts
16. impairment	35. behavioral	53. psychotic	72. expectancies
17. distress	36. cognitive-behavioral	54. cannabis	73. behaviors
18. sedating		55. perception	
19. organs	37. Alcoholics Anonymous	56. bodily	
20. medical		57. behavioral	

MULTIPLE CHOICE

1. (d) is correct. (a) is the physiological response to discontinued use of alcohol; (b) the temporary state occasioned by alcohol use; and (c) is the combined effect of two or more psychoactive substances.
2. (b) is correct. All of the other choices are associated with the rate of alcohol absorption.
3. (a) is correct. There is no support for (b), (c), or (d).
4. (a) is correct. Disufiram, also known as Antabuse, inhibits the enzyme aldehyde dehydrogenase (d); (b) makes alcohol less reinforcing; and (c) is sometimes combined with disulfiram.
5. (b) is correct. (a), (c), and (d) are not correct.
6. (c) is correct. (a), (b), and (d) do not refer to this effect.
7. (d) is correct. There is no support for (a), (b), or (c).
8. (a) is correct. Other drugs belong to the classes named in (b), (c), and (d).
9. (d) is correct. There is no support for (a), (b), or (c).
10. (a) is correct. There is no support for (b), (c), or (d).
11. (d) is correct. (a) is an in-patient setting where patient and health-care providers work closely together; (b) is a residential setting combining community living arrangements, work, and therapy; and (c) is a 12-step support group.
12. (a) is correct. There is no support for (b), (c), or (d).
13. (c) is correct. (a) is the need for more of a substance to achieve the desired effect; (b) is a temporary state occasioned by substance use; and (d) is the combined effect of two or more psychoactive substances.
14. (d) is correct. (a) is one effect of a certain type of psychoactive substance; (b) is sometimes used to mean the same thing as intoxication; (c) is the body's breakdown and processing of any ingested substance.
15. (d) is correct. (a) is not necessarily associated with dementia; (b) and (c) are forms of dementia not related to

alcohol use.

16. (d) is correct. (a), (b), and (c) would undermine her abstinence efforts.
17. (a) is correct. (b), (c), and (d) are not spiritually based.
18. (d) is correct. Other psychoactive substances affect (a), (b), and (c).
19. (c) is correct. (a), (b), and (d) may be associated with the use of a hallucinogen.
20. (a) is correct. (b) and (c) are synthetic psychoactive substances; and there is no evidence for (d).
21. (b) is correct. (a) involves a decreased sensitivity to the substance; (c) to the physiological reaction of not ingesting the substance; and (d) to using a substance in spite of ill effects.
22. (b) is correct. (a) is associated with dependence; (c) with tolerance; and (d) with craving.
23. (d) is correct. (a) involves continued use of drugs despite risks or problems in living; (b) is using drugs to achieve a mood or physical state; and (c) usage of increased amounts to achieve the same result.
24. (c) is correct. (a) is another form of dementia; (b) is not a disorder; and (d) is a tic and motor disorder.
25. (b) is correct. There is no evidence for (a), (c), and (d).
26. (a) is correct. (b), (c), and (d) are not necessarily associated with alcohol.
27. (c) is correct. (d) is methadone; there is no medication to treat alcoholism, as such (a), though medications are used to treat some symptoms; and (b) is a substance used to cause an aversive biological response to drinking alcohol.
28. (d) is correct. (a) is not related to drug use; (b) is a symptom involved in withdrawal from alcohol; and (c) is a form of dementia associated with prolonged alcohol use.
29. (b) is correct. (c) is the most widely abused legal substance; (d) is a legal substance; (a) is popular but not as widely used as marijuana.
30. (d) is correct. (a) and (b) natural pain-killing substances produced by the brain; and (c) is an opioid similar to heroin.

CHAPTER **14**
EATING DISORDERS AND
IMPULSE-CONTROL DISORDERS

CHAPTER AT A GLANCE

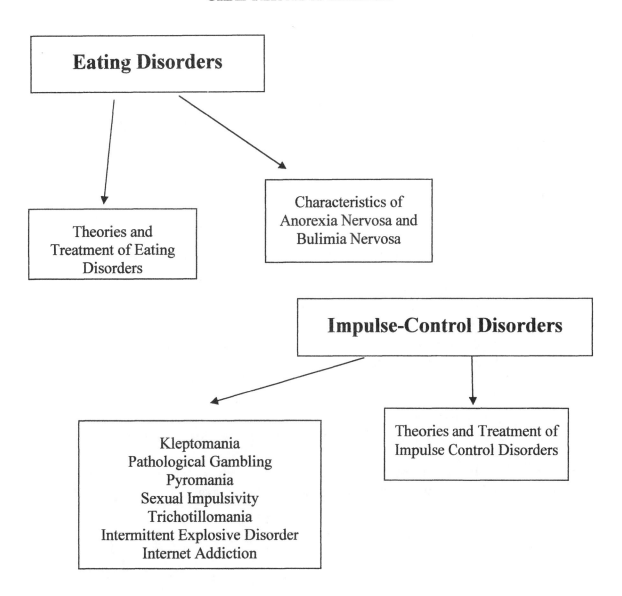

Learning Objectives

1.0   Eating Disorders
    1.1   Indicate the characteristics of anorexia nervosa.
    1.2   Identify the features of bulimia nervosa.
    1.3   Compare and contrast the theories and treatments of eating disorders.
2.0   The Nature of Impulse Control Disorders
    2.1   Identify the essential features common to the impulse control disorders.
3.0   Kleptomania
    3.1   Summarize the characteristics of kleptomania.
    3.2   Indicate the relevant theories and treatments of kleptomania.
4.0   Pathological Gambling
    4.1   Describe the symptoms of pathological gambling.
    4.2   Contrast the theoretical perspectives used to understand and treat pathological gambling.
5.0   Pyromania
    5.1   Indicate the diagnostic features of pyromania.
    5.2   Discuss theories and treatments of pyromania.
6.0   Sexual Impulsivity
    6.1   Outline the characteristic behaviors associated with sexual impulsivity.
    6.2   Indicate the theoretical understanding and treatment of sexual impulsivity.
7.0   Trichotillomania
    7.1   Describe the symptoms used to diagnose trichotillomania.
    7.2   Compare perspectives to understanding and treating the disorder.
8.0   Intermittent Explosive Disorder
    8.1   Summarize the features of intermittent explosive disorder.
    8.2   Describe relevant theories and treatments.
9.0   Internet Addiction
    9.1   Summarize the features of Internet addiction.
    9.2   Describe relevant theories and treatments.
10.0   Eating Disorders and Impulse Control Disorders: The Biopsychosocial Perspective
11.0   Chapter Boxes
    11.1   Discuss the case of actress Tracey Gold.
    11.2   Indicate the issues involved in the widespread availability of legalized gambling.

Identifying Treatments

For each of the disorders listed below, identify the psychological treatments (behavioral, cognitive, etc.) that are used:

1. Eating disorders

   _____

2. Kleptomania

   _____

3. Pathological Gambling

   _____

4. Pyromania

   _____

5. Sexual Impulsivity

   _____

6. Trichotillmania

   _____

Matching

Put the letter from the right-hand column corresponding to the correct match in the blank next to each item in the left-hand column.

1. ____ Neurotransmitter system thought to play a role in the development of kleptomania, pyromania, intermittent explosive disorder, and eating disorders.
2. ____ Physical disorder thought to be linked to intermittent explosive disorder.
3. ____ Type of bulimia nervosa in which the individual tries to force out of the body excess food taken in during a binge by vomiting or using laxatives.
4. ____ Hormone that may be present in unusually high levels in individuals with sexual impulsivity.
5. ____ Psychiatrist who established the first U.S. clinic for treatment of pathological gambling.
6. ____ Axis II disorder thought to be linked to eating disorder.
7. ____ Well-known sports figure who was publicly exposed as a pathological gambler.
8. ____ Medication found to be effective in reducing kleptomanic behavior.
9. ____ Type of bulimia nervosa in which the individual tries to compensate for binges by engaging in fasting or excessive exercise.
10. ____ Bet that results in a large amount of money and is influential in propelling an individual to become a pathological gambler.
11. ____ Serial murderer, also known as "Son of Sam," who set more than 2000 fires in New York City during the 1970s.
12. ____ Psychological disorder thought to be linked to trichotillomania.

a. testosterone
b. Robert Custer
c. obsessive-compulsive disorder
d. big win
e. Pete Rose
f. serotonin
g. nonpurging type
h. fluoxetine
i. David Berkowitz
j. borderline personality disorder
k. purging type
l. epilepsy

Word Scramble Puzzle

This puzzle is like the popular word game in which players form words from tiles that each has a certain value. The following letters are the ones in your "pile" with their assigned values. These letters can be combined in different ways to form the words described in the clues at the left. When you arrange the letters correctly, you will have the point value listed in parentheses. You can use each letter more than once to solve the clues.

Letter	Value	Letter	Value	Letter	Value	Letter	Value
A	1	H	4	N	1	T	1
B	3	I	1	O	1	U	1
C	3	K	5	P	3	V	4
E	1	L	1	R	1	X	8
G	2	M	3	S	1	Y	4

1. An impulse-control disorder characterized by a persistent and compelling urge to start fires _____ (16 points).
2. An impulse-control disorder involving the persistent urge to steal _____ (19 points).
3. In intermittent _____ disorder, the individual experiences uncontrollable violent bursts of anger (21 points).
4. In the eating disorder _____ nervosa, the individual has a view of herself as overweight, even though she may be near starvation (15 points).
5. The behavior engaged by individuals with eating disorders when they attempt to rid themselves of food they have already eaten _____ (11 points).
6. In _____ nervosa, the individual may maintain a normal weight, though she yields to uncontrollable urges to overeat and then rid herself of what she has eaten (11 points).
7. An uncontrollable urge to act is called an _____ (11 points).
8. An impulse-control disorder involving the uncontrollable and compulsive urge to pull out one's hair _____ (23 points).

Short Answer

1. What are three essential features of the behavior of people with an impulse-control disorder?

_____

_____

2. For each of the following disorders, describe a somatic treatment found to be helpful in reducing symptoms and the proposed mechanism of action of this treatment:

Disorder	Somatic treatment	Mechanism of action
Kleptomania		
Sexual impulsivity		
Trichotillomania		

Disorder	Somatic treatment	Mechanism of action
Intermittent explosive disorder		
Eating disorders		

3. What are the two key differences between anorexia nervosa and bulimia nervosa?

_____

_____

4. Describe the role of faulty cognitions in the development of pathological gambling and eating disorders:

Disorder	Role of faulty cognitions
Pathological gambling	
Eating disorders	

5. What three lines of evidence regarding the relationship between mood disorders and impulse control disorders support the contention that these disorders are on the same "affective spectrum"?

_____

_____

_____

6. Summarize the main features of each of the following stages involved in the development of pathological gambling:

Stage	Main features
Recreational gambling	
Early winning stage	
The big win	
Chasing	
Establishment of pathological gambling cycle	

7. Describe the hypothesized role of family relationships in the development or maintenance of the following disorders:

Disorder	Role of family relationships
Pathological gambling	
Sexual impulsivity	
Trichotillomania	
Eating disorders	

From the Case Files of Dr. Sarah Tobin: Thinking About Rosa's Case

Answer the following questions about the case of Rosa Nomirez.

1. Describe how Rosa's symptoms met the diagnostic criteria for anorexia nervosa.

_____

_____

2. What was Dr. Tobin's case formulation for Rosa's diagnosis of anorexia nervosa?

_____

_____

3. Discuss the nature and course of Rosa's treatment.

_____

_____

4. How did Dr. Tobin respond to Rosa's refusal to participate in group therapy?

_____

_____

Focusing on Research

Answer the following questions from the text box "How People Differ: Does Modern Society Cause Eating Disorders?"

1. Comment on the pattern of eating disorders in African-American and Caucasian women in the United States.

_____

_____

2. What possible explanations are there to explain the relative infrequency of eating disorders in non-Western cultures?

_____

_____

3. What individual characteristics may contribute to eating disorders?

_____

_____

Review at a Glance

Test your knowledge by completing the blank spaces with terms from the chapter. If you need a hint, consult the chapter summary.

People with anorexia nervosa show four kinds of symptoms. They refuse or are unable to (1) _____; have an intense fear of (2) _____ or (3) _____; have a (4) _____ perception of their (5) _____ or _____; and experience (6) _____, if they are post-puberty. People with bulimia nervosa alternate between (7)_____ and (8)_____. Biological explanations for eating disorders focus on abnormalities in the (9) _____ and (10) _____ neurotransmitter systems. The psychological perspective sees people who have eating disorders as suffering from a great deal of (11) _____ and as turning to food for (12) _____ and (13) _____. Cognitive theories focus on the client's (14) _____ and resistance to (15) _____. Sociocultural explanations emphasize both the (16) _____ system and society's attitudes toward (17) _____ and (18) _____. Interventions include (19) _____, individual (20)_____, (21)_____ and (22)_____ techniques, and (23)_____ therapy.

People with (24) _____ disorders repeatedly engage in behaviors that are potentially harmful, and they feel unable (25) _____ and a sense of (26) _____ if they are thwarted in their desires. People with (27) _____ are driven by a persistent urge to steal because they experience a (28) _____ while engaging in stealing. Treatments include medication, usually (29) _____, and (30) _____ treatments, such as (31) _____.

(32)_____ have an intense urge to gamble. Biological factors can be seen as a drive for (33) _____ and (34) _____ feelings. Certain personality characteristics, such as (35) _____ and (36) _____, also predispose people to develop this condition. Sociocultural factors, such as the spread of (37) _____, may aggravate some people's tendencies to become immersed in such behavior. Treatments include medications, such as (38) _____, which are helpful, as are (39) _____ and (40) _____ techniques. Many pathological gamblers also benefit from participation in peer groups, such as (41) _____.

People with (42) _____ have an intense desire to prepare, set, and watch (43) _____. This disorder seems rooted in (44) _____ problems and (45) _____ behavior. Adults with pyromania typically have problems with (46) _____ and (47) _____. Interventions aimed at adults are designed to address the client's (48)

_____, (49) _____, (50) _____ problems, and inability to control (51) _____.

People with (52) _____ are unable to control their sexual behavior. Individuals with this condition commonly suffer coexisting conditions, such as (53) _____, (54) _____ disorder, (55) _____, or some (56) _____ symptoms. Treatment usually combines (57) _____ -oriented, (58) _____, and (59) _____ systems approaches.

People with (60) _____ have an irresistible urge to pull out their hair. This condition is associated with (61) _____ disorders, (62) _____ abnormalities, disturbed (63) _____ relationships, and the fact that the behavior relieves (64) _____. The most common intervention is a form of (65) _____ therapy, aimed at (66) _____.

People with (67) _____ disorder feel an inability to resist assaultive or destructive acts of (68) _____, caused by an interaction of (69) _____ and (70) _____ factors. Treatment may involve both (71) _____ and (72) _____.

Multiple Choice

1. During the course of committing an impulsive act, people with impulse-control disorders
   a. usually feel tension and anxiety immediately after engaging in the impulsive act.
   b. may experience arousal before engaging in the impulsive act that they liken to sexual excitement.
   c. feel intensely conflicted at the moment of choosing to engage in the impulsive act.
   d. often experience feelings of regret and remorse immediately before engaging in the impulsive act.

2. Which of the following statements is true regarding people with kleptomania?
   a. They are driven by a desire to accumulate expensive possessions.
   b. They limit their stealing to situations in which they are taking items from people whom they know personally.
   c. They are driven by the desire to steal, not the desire to have.
   d. They rarely suffer from psychological disorders other than the problem of kleptomania.

3. Researchers investigating the role of biological factors in pathological gambling have found that these individuals
   a. show more norepinephrine activity than nongamblers.
   b. have thyroid abnormalities.
   c. have lower levels of dopamine than nongamblers.
   d. show evidence of specific biological markers.

4. A treatment of pathological gambling involving clients imagining scenes in which they feel tempted to gamble and relaxing as they imagine each successive behavior involved in the scene is called
   a. covert sensitization.
   b. flooding.
   c. *in vivo* desensitization.
   d. imaginal desensitization.

5. The type of bulimia nervosa in which one rids the body of food with vomiting, laxatives, or diuretics is
   a. anorexic.
   b. purging.
   c. depressive.
   d. nonpurging.

6. According to government estimates, the highest rates for legalized gambling occur in which states?.
   a. casinos are built in expensive resort areas
   b. gambling has been legalized for many years.
   c. there are lotteries but not casinos.
   d. new casinos and lotteries have been developed.

7. Prior to engaging in a seemingly uncontrollable act, people with intermittent explosive disorder experience a phenomenon similar to that experienced by people with
   a. epilepsy.
   b. high blood pressure.
   c. cardiovascular disease.
   d. migraine headache disorder

8. Research on the relationship between dieting and eating disorders indicates that
   a. dieters are at lower risk for developing eating disorders.
   b. there is no relationship between dieting and eating disorders.
   c. dieters are at greater risk for developing eating disorders.
   d. exercisers, but not dieters, are likely to develop eating disorders.

9. Proponents of which theoretical model propose that people with bulimia translate society's attitudes toward thinness into extreme restraints and rigid rules about food?
   a. biological
   b. psychodynamic
   c. family systems
   d. cognitive-behavioral

10. Extreme cases of sexual impulsivity are sometimes treated biologically with
    a. antiandrogenic medication.
    b. testosterone.
    c. ECT.
    d. neuroleptics.

11. According to Custer's views regarding the development of pathological gambling, the transition to becoming a pathological gambler becomes evident when the gambler:
    a. starts to gain an identity as a winner.
    b. starts to develop fears of becoming a loser.
    c. begins to experience family problems.
    d. seeks professional help for the gambling problem.

12. The Goldfarb Fear of Fat Scale would be used in the diagnosis of
    a. bulimia nervosa.
    b. anorexia nervosa.
    c. eating disorders involving possible medical complications.
    d. any eating disorder.

13. Which behavioral technique involves having the individual with kleptomania imagine disgusting images, such as vomit, when the compulsion to steal is beginning?
    a. free association
    b. flooding
    c. covert sensitization
    d. *in vivo* desensitization

14. Which of the following techniques involves having the client with pyromania construct a chart that corresponds to the individual's behaviors, feelings, and experiences associated with firesetting?
    a. the graphing technique
    b. the thought stopping technique
    c. aversive conditioning
    d. *in vivo* desensitization

15. According to the family systems perspective, adults with sexual impulsivity are more likely to grow up in families with
    a. restrictive attitudes regarding sex.
    b. permissive attitudes regarding sex.
    c. liberal opinions regarding sex.
    d. open attitudes about sex

16. Trichotillomania is an impulse-control disorder involving the persistent urge to
    a. pull one's hair.
    b. bite one's nails.
    c. binge, then purge.
    d. engage in sexual intercourse.

17. While stopped in his car at a stoplight, Tim occasionally experiences an aura, followed by an intense urge to get out of the car and pummel the person in the car ahead of him for no apparent reason. He has been arrested several times for acting on this urge. What impulse-control disorder might Tim suffer from?
    a. antisocial personality disorder
    b. oppositional defiant disorder
    c. intermittent explosive disorder
    d. passive aggressive personality disorder

18. Which of the following is considered to be the core feature of anorexia nervosa?
    a. frequent binging
    b. normal body weight
    c. consumption of nonnutritive substances
    d. body image disturbance

19. The highest rates for anorexia nervosa are found in
    a. China.
    b. France.
    c. India.
    d. the United States

20. Which of the following facts might support a conclusion that an individual's gambling behavior was beyond the boundaries of social gambling?
    a. He was seeking a big win.
    b. He started drinking while he was gambling.
    c. His wife approved of his gambling.
    d. He promised his wife that he would stop but did not.

21. Which of the following is one of the main differences between anorexics and bulimics?
    a. Anorexics are comfortable with their body image; bulimics are not.
    b. Anorexics are typically overweight; bulimics are typically underweight.
    c. Anorexics have a normal body weight; bulimics are typically overweight.
    d. Anorexics have a distorted body image; bulimics generally do not.

22. Family systems theorists view the anorexic behavior of the teenage girl as being an effort to
    a. assert her independence.
    b. express her concerns.
    c. modify her position in the family structure.
    d. reduce anxiety.

23. Which medication reduces the symptoms of bulimia by increasing serotonin levels?
    a. Prozac
    b. Halcion
    c. Mellaril
    d. Ritalin

24 Anne has a persistent urge to shoplift. However, her motivation for stealing is not based in need. She steals for the sake of fulfilling her impulse to do so. Which impulse-control disorder might she be diagnosed as having?
    a. antisocial personality disorder
    b. pyromania
    c. trichotillomania
    d. kleptomania

25 The gain of a large amount of money in one bet through which a compulsive gambler becomes propelled into a pattern of gambling is referred to as the
    a. jackpot.
    b. big stakes.
    c. big win.
    d. obsession.

26 The impulse-control disorder characterized by a persistent urge to start fires is called
    a. kleptomania.
    b. rumination disorder.
    c. trichotillomania.
    d. pyromania.

27. According to family theorists, childhood neglect and abuse may result in which impulse control disorder?
    a. anorexia nervosa
    b. kleptomania
    c. sexual impulsivity
    d. bulimia nervosa

28. Andrea is an 8-year-old girl who compulsively pulls her hair out and occasionally eats it. She continues this behavior despite the fact that she has very noticeable bald spots. Which impulse-control disorder might she have?
    a. intermittent explosive disorder
    b. stereotypy/habit disorder
    c. pica
    d. trichotillomania

Answers

IDENTIFYING TREATMENTS

1. Self-monitoring, self-control strategies, problem solving techniques, cognitive restructuring, helping client cope with stress in interpersonal situations, enhanced self-esteem, and group therapy or family therapy.
2. Covert sensitization, thought stopping.
3. Training in problem solving, correcting inaccurate perceptions of gambling, training in social skills, relapse prevention, and Gamblers Anonymous.
4. Outreach and community prevention, prevention programs for children and adolescents, enhanced self-esteem, family therapy, and group or individual therapy based on behavioral, cognitive or psychodynamic model.
5. Bringing to surface underlying conflicts that motivate behavior, aversive covert conditioning, imaginal desensitization, behavioral contracting, and family or couples therapy.
6. Habit reversal (i.e. substitute alternative behaviors for the impulsive act); social support.

MATCHING

1. f	4. a	7. e	10. d
2. l	5. b	8. h	11. i
3. k	6. j	9. g	12. c

WORD SCRAMBLE

1. PYROMANIA	4. ANOREXIA	7. IMPULSE
2. KLEPTOMANIA	5. PURGING	8. TRICHOTILLOMANIA
3. EXPLOSIVE	6. BULIMIA	

SHORT ANSWER

1.
They are unable to stop from acting on impulses that are harmful to self or others.
Before they act on their impulse, they feel pressured to act.
Upon acting on their impulse, they feel a sense of pleasure or gratification similar to sexual release.

2.

Disorder	Somatic treatment	Mechanism of action
Kleptomania	Fluoxetine (Prozac)	Increases availability of serotonin
Sexual impulsivity	Antiandrogenic medication	Reduces level of testosterone
Trichotillomania	Lithium	Not described in text.
	Clomipramine	Antidepressant that reduces obsessional symptoms.
Intermittent explosive disorder	Benzodiazepines	Used to reduce explosive behavior in people with certain personality disorders.
	Lithium	Both reduce emotional reactivity by lowering norepinephrine functioning.
	Beta blockers	
Eating disorders	Fluoxetine	Increases availability of serotonin.

231

Disorder	Somatic treatment	Mechanism of action
	Antidepressants	Reduce depressive symptoms and reduce eating disorder behaviors specifically.
	MAO inhibitors	No longer used because of undesirable side effects.

3. **Body image**: People with anorexia nervosa see themselves as overweight no matter how emaciated they may be; people with bulimia nervosa have normal body image.
   Amount of weight loss: People with anorexia nervosa are significantly below the norm for weight; people with bulimia are of normal or above average weight.

4.

Disorder	Role of faulty cognitions
Pathological gambling	Pathological gamblers hold faulty beliefs that they are in control of the probabilities that affect the outcome of their bets; this leads them to develop grandiose ideas that lead them to become convinced of their ultimate success.
Eating disorders	The individual's incorporation of society's beliefs about thinness leads the individual to adopt a set of rules and restrictions regarding food; in the case of bulimia nervosa, these rules break down when the individual becomes hungry, and a binge pattern is set in motion.

5.
a. Several impulse-control disorders have been found to co-occur with mood disorders including kleptomania, pathological gambling, and eating disorders. Trichotillomania is thought to be linked to obsessive-compulsive disorder, another disorder that would fall on a proposed affective spectrum.
b. Altered functioning of serotonin and norepinephrine neurotransmitters, systems that are thought to play a role in mood disorders, has been observed in people with impulse-control disorders including kleptomania, pathological gambling, pyromania, and eating disorders.
c. Treatments used for mood disorders have been successfully applied to the impulse-control disorders: kleptomania, trichotillomania, intermittent explosive disorder, and eating disorders.

6.

Stage	Main features
Recreational gambling	The person's behavior is indistinguishable from that of a gambler who enjoys gambling as a social activity.
Early winning stage	The individual begins to win and starts to gain gambling skills. Development of identity as a "winner"occurs, and through continued wins, that identity becomes reinforced.
The big win	A gain of a large amount of money in one bet is so highly reinforcing that the individual becomes possessed with the need to re-experience it. The gambler is convinced of the possession of unique luck and skill and starts to make riskier bets.
Chasing	After losses inevitably start to occur, the individual begins to bet more and more to recoup earlier losses. As desperation mounts, the individual is launched into an intensive and all-consuming enterprise. Poor judgment combined with desperation lead to larger and larger losses.

Stage	Main features
Establishment of pathological gambling cycle	In a continued search for another big win, the individual has periodic wins that maintain his or her unreasonable optimism. In time, however, the individual's resources become depleted, and the person may consider drastic action such as suicide, running away, or a life of crime to support the behavior.

7.

Disorder	Role of family relationships
Pathological gambling	Spouses and children of pathological gamblers are affected by the disorder. Spouses report detrimental changes in emotional functioning; dysfunctional coping behaviors; emotional, verbal, or physical abuse; and feelings of suicidality. Children experience significant behavioral and adjustment problems in school and at home and involvement in drug or alcohol abuse, crime, or gambling-related activities. Families also suffer financially due to heavy betting expenses.
Sexual impulsivity	The disorder is thought to result from either unduly restrictive attitudes toward sex in a child's family or childhood neglect and abuse. The disorder may result in or be maintained in adulthood by dysfunctional communication patterns in the sexual domain between sexual partners.
Trichotillomania	Described in terms of psychodynamic theory, disturbed parent-child relationships are thought to create feelings of neglect, abandonment, or emotional burdening in a child who attempts to gain attention or gratification through hair-pulling.
Eating disorders	Family systems theorists propose that a girl may develop anorexia nervosa in an effort to assert her independence from the family, perhaps in situations where the girl feels that her parents are standing in the way of her becoming autonomous. Other contributing factors may be a family that is chaotic, incapable of resolving conflict, unaffectionate, and lacking in empathy.

FROM THE CASE FILES OF DR. SARAH TOBIN: THINKING ABOUT ROSA'S CASE

1. Her MMPI-2 profile showed her to be defensive, hypersensitive, depressive, and a perfectionist—features commonly associated with eating disorders. She had lost nearly 20 percent of her body weight in the past several months, had stopped menstruating, and had showed signs of anemia, dehydration, and electrolyte disturbance. She had an intense fear of gaining weight, even though she was drastically underweight, and she had a disturbed perception of her body weight and figure.
2. Her problems went back to childhood, when her parents became overprotective of her after the death of her brother at the age of 5. Her parents expected a lot of her, and she did not want to disappoint them. She strove for perfection in every area of her life, but when she began college, she feared that she would not meet the expectations of her parents and others. As her self-doubts increased, she developed distorted concepts of her intelligence, personality, and attractiveness. She stopped eating in an effort to become more attractive. At 117 pounds, she thought she was fat.
3. Rosa developed a nutritional and meal plan with a nutritionist and had individual therapy with Dr. Tobin for 6 months. Dr. Tobin used mainly cognitive techniques to help Rosa develop more accurate views of herself, the world, and her potential. She complied with the medical treatment and improved in all areas of her life. She was able to talk to her parents about her need to feel less pressure from them, and she survived the tennis team's loss of the championship.
4. Dr. Tobin was sensitive to the fact that, in the Puerto Rican culture, seeking help for psychological problems carried a great stigma. She understood Rosa's insistence that she could not talk about her problem with peers.

FOCUSING ON RESEARCH

1. Within the United States, eating disorders are far less prevalent among African American women compared with Caucasian women, and a similar pattern holds true for specific symptoms such as restrictive dieting and body image distortion.
2. The ideal body image for a woman, according to the American cultural ideal, is tied to thinness. Over the past several decades, the ideal woman has gotten thinner and thinner. At the same time, the average body mass and height of women has increased (perhaps due to improvements in health and nutrition), making the cultural ideal increasingly difficult to obtain. There is evidence that, as women from other cultures adopt Western standards of beauty, restrictive dieting eating disorders becomes more prevalent.
3. Men and women with personality characteristics of perfectionism, obsessiveness, or a sense of personal ineffectiveness and people with biological predispositions and problems in psychosocial development may be more prone to eating disorders.

REVIEW AT A GLANCE

1. maintain normal weight
2. gaining weight
3. becoming fat
4. distorted
5. weight; shape
6. amenorrhea
7. binging
8. purging
9. norepinephrine
10. serotonin
11. inner turmoil
12. comfort
13. nurturance
14. rigidity
15. change
16. family
17. eating
18. diet
19. medication
20. therapy
21. cognitive-behavioral
22. interpersonal
23. family
24. impulse control
25. stop themselves
26. desperation
27. kleptomania
28. thrill
29. fluoxetine
30. behavioral
31. covert sensitization
32. Pathological gamblers
33. stimulation
34. pleasurable
35. impulsivity
36. psychopathy
37. legalized gambling
38. selective serotonin reuptake inhibitors
39. behavioral
40. cognitive-behavioral
41. Gamblers Anonymous
42. pyromania
43. fires
44. childhood
45. firesetting
46. substance abuse
47. relationship difficulties
48. low self-esteem
49. depression
50. communication
51. anger
52. sexual impulsivity
53. depression
54. phobic
55. substance abuse
56. dissociative
57. insight
58. behavioral
59. family
60. trichotillomania
61. obsessive-compulsive
62. brain
63. parent-child
64. tension
65. behavior
66. habit reversal
67. intermittent explosive
68. aggression
69. biological
70. environmental
71. medication
72. psychotherapy

MULTIPLE CHOICE

1. (b) is correct. They do not feel either (a), (c), or (d).
2. (c) is correct. (a), (b), and (d) are not true.
3. (a) is correct. There is no evidence for the existence of (b), (c), and (d).
4. (d) is correct. a) involves imagining others condoning one's actions; (b) is a type of therapy in which the client experiences an intense form of her phobia or other undesirable object/event; (c) involves therapy in the actual problem situation.
5. (b) is correct. (a) does not involve binging and purging; (c) is not a form of bulimia, and ; (d) is a type of bulimia that does not involve eliminating the contents of consumption from one's body.
6. (b) is correct. There is no evidence for (a), (c), or (d).
7. (a) is correct. There is no evidence of (b), (c), or (d).
8. (c) is correct. (a) and (b) are false, in fact the opposite is usually true; there is not evidence for (d).
9. (c) is correct. (a) is not a theoretical model; (b) believes that childhood experience and intrapsychic conflict are

contributing to the disorder; (c) that dysfunctional family dynamics play a role.
10. (a) is correct. (b) may increase sexual desire; (c) and (d) would not be used as treatment.
11. (a) is correct. (b), (c), and (d) have nothing to do with increasing gambling behavior.
12. (b) is correct. The scale is not used with (a), (c), or (d).
13. (c) is correct. (a) is a psychodynamic therapy technique; (b) and (d) involve real situations.
14. (a) is correct. (b), (c), and (d) do not involve charting behavior.
15. (a) is correct. (b), (c), and (d) may mitigate against sexual impulsivity.
16. (a) is correct. (b) and (d) are not impulse-control disorders; (c) is bulimia nervosa.
17. (c) is correct. (a) could account for violent acts, but not as described; (b) and (d) are not generally associated with violence and out-of-control behavior.
18. (d) is correct. (a) is a factor of bulimia, not anorexia; (b) is definitely not a factor in anorexia; (c) is related to a disorder known as pica.
19. (d) is correct. Rates are much lower in (a), (b), and (c) than in (d).
20. (d) is correct. (a), (b), and (c) may contribute to the behaviors, but (d) indicates that it is becoming addictive.
21. (d) is correct. (a), (b), and (c) are all incorrect comparisons.
22. (a) is correct. (b), (c), and (d) are not considered factors in the development of anorexia nervosa.
23. (a) is correct. (b), (c), and (d) do not affect serotonin levels and are not used to treat bulimia.
24. (d) is correct. (a) is a disorder associated with criminal behavior and violations of rights of others; (b) with firesetting; and (c) with pulling out one's hair.
25. (c) is correct. (a) may be the source of a large payoff; (b) has to do with what one has wagered; and (d) is an intrusive thought.
26. (d) is correct. (a) is compulsive stealing; (b) regurgitating food; and (c) pulling out one's hair.
27. (c) is correct. Childhood abuse has not been linked to (a), (b), or (d).
28. (d) is correct. (a) is uncontrolled violent outbursts; (b) a repetitive behavior; and (c) eating nonfood items.

CHAPTER **15**
ETHICAL AND LEGAL ISSUES

CHAPTER AT A GLANCE

Ethical and Legal Issues

Roles and Responsibilities of Clinicians
Therapist Competence
Informed Consent
Confidentiality
Relationships with Client
The Business of Psychotherapy
Special Roles for Clinicians

Commitment
Right to Refuse Treatment
Refusal of Treatment

Forensic Issues
Insanity Defense
Competency to Stand Trial

Learning Objectives

1.0   Ethical Issues
     1.1   Identify the roles and responsibilities of mental health clinicians and the notion of therapist competence.
     1.2   Describe the concept of informed consent and discuss its relevance to psychological treatment.
     1.3   Explain the importance of confidentiality and the related concept of privileged communication, and discuss the exceptions to these principles, such as the duty to warn.
     1.4   Discuss the nature of a clinician's relationships with clients.
     1.5   Outline the major concerns of the business of psychotherapy.
     1.6   Distinguish the special roles clinicians may play, including that of an expert legal witness, a *guardian ad litem*, evaluator in child protection cases, and conducting evaluations of being with symptoms of cognitive decline.
     1.7   Discuss the process of involuntary commitment as a means of protecting the client and others from the expression of dangerous behaviors, including the principle of *parens patriae*.
     1.8   Indicate the importance of the client's right to treatment and a humane environment, liberty, and safety.
     1.9   Describe the client's right to refuse treatment and to live in the least restrictive alternative to an institution.

2.0   Forensic Issues in Psychological Treatment
     2.1   Discuss the general nature of the work of forensic psychologists.
     2.2   Explain the insanity defense and the role of the forensic psychologist in its use.
     2.3   Discuss the history of the insanity defense, from its beginnings in Great Britain to the enactment of the Insanity Defense Reform Act of 1984.
     ~~2.4~~   Compare and contrast the relevance and outcomes of the insanity defenses in the cases of John Hinckley, Jeffrey Dahmer, Erik and Lyle Menendez, Lorena Bobbitt, Theodore Kacznyski, Lee Boyd Malvo, and John Allen Muhammed.
     2.5   Describe how and why competency to stand trial becomes an issue in criminal proceedings and discuss the role of forensic psychologists in its use.

3.0   Chapter Box
     ~~3.1~~   Discuss the case of John Hinckley.

Matching

Put the letter from the right-hand column corresponding to the correct match in the blank next to each item in the left-hand column.

1. ____ Responsibility of a clinician to warn a person of possible threat or danger presented by client's behavior.

2. ____ Evaluation of a client's ability to participate in court proceedings on behalf of his or her own defense.

3. ____ Protection of information about a client obtained in the process of providing treatment.

4. ____ Need to "appreciate" the wrongfulness of an act.

5. ____ Proof of "insanity" needed.

6. ____ Legal procedure designed to protect individuals incapable of doing so such as a minor or incapacitated adult.

7. ____ Appointed by a court to make decisions privileged for a person.

8. ____ Client's participation in setting, understanding, and agreeing to treatment goals.
9. ____ Treatment setting that provides the fewest constraints on a client's freedom.
10. ____ Legal requirement that professionals notify appropriate authorities about cases in which children and other vulnerable individuals are being abused.
11. ____ Authority of the state to protect those who are unable to protect themselves.
12. ____ Information provided by a client to a clinician that cannot be disclosed in court without the client's permission.

a. confidentiality
b. duty to warn
c. competency to stand trial
d. Insanity Defense Reform Act
e. ALI
f. informed consent
g. Least Restrictive environment
h. guardian ad litem
i. mandated reporting
j. privileged communication
k. parens patriae
l. committment

Short Answer

1. Answer each of the following questions about forensic issues in psychological treatment.

   a. Why was there a difference between the outcome of the Jeffrey Dahmer case and that of the John Hinckley case?

   _____

   _____

   b. What have been the major issues identified in legislation and judicial rulings regarding the definition of insanity?

   _____

   _____

   c. What factors are assessed in determining a person's competency to stand trial?

   _____

   _____

   d. How do clinicians attempt to balance the need to commit a person involuntarily to treatment against the individual's right to the least restrictive alternative?

   _____

   _____

   e. What issues are involved in a clinician's protecting a client's confidentiality versus the need to notify potential victims of harm?

   _____

   _____

f. What are the basic components of treatment to which hospitalized clients are entitled by law?

_____

_____

2. Answer the following pursuant to the Guidelines for Psychological Evaluations in Child Protection Matters.

    a. The primary purpose of the evaluation is:

    _____

    _____

    b. Whose interests and well-being are paramount?

    _____

    _____

    c. The evaluation addresses:

    _____

    _____

    d. What do the guidelines mandate about reporting on the psychological functioning of any individual?

    _____

    _____

    e. What must be the basis for any recommendations made by the psychologist?

    _____

    _____

3. Answer the following concerning the Guidelines for the Evaluation of Dementia and Age-Related Cognitive Decline.

    a. What must the psychologist at least attempt to obtain before beginning the evaluation of a person with dementia or age-related cognitive decline?

    _____

    _____

    b. What assessment procedures should be used if possible?

    _____

    _____

    c. What should the examiner attempt to provide in addition to conducting an assessment?

    _____

    _____

    _____

4. Answer the following from "Social Context: Homeless and Mentally Ill: The Right to Refuse Treatment."

    a. State the evidence that homeless people with schizophrenia experience more severe symptoms than those who are not homeless.

    _____

    _____

b. What aspect of medication is cited as one reason for widespread homelessness among people with schizophrenia?

_____

_____

c. What do we need to know about the relationship between homelessness and noncompliance with medication for schizophrenia?

_____

_____

Focusing on Research

Answer the following questions from "Research Focus: The Prediction of Violent Behavior."

1. What is the single best predictor of violence?

_____

_____

2. Discuss the problems inherent in psychologists' attempts to predict a person's behavior.

_____

_____

3. Summarize the guidelines for psychologists' prediction of violence suggested by forensic psychologist John Monahan.

_____

_____

From the Case Files of Dr. Sarah Tobin: Thinking About Mark's Case

Answer the following questions about the case of Mark Chen.

1. Why did Dr. Tobin have no choice but to ask Tanya to commit Mark involuntarily to the hospital?

_____

_____

2. Discuss Dr. Tobin's assessment and diagnosis of Mark.

_____

_____

3. What was Dr. Tobin's formulation of Mark's case?

_____

_____

4. Describe the nature and course of Mark's treatment.

_____

_____

Review at a Glance

Test your knowledge by completing the blank spaces with terms from the chapter. If you need a hint, consult the chapter summary.

Clinicians are expected to have the intellectual competence to (1) _____, (2) _____, and (3) _____ clients whom they accept into treatment. When beginning work with clients, they should obtain the client's (4) _____ to ensure that the client understands the (5) _____ of treatment, the process of (6) _____, the client's (7) _____, the therapist's (8) _____, treatment (9) _____, (10) _____ that will be used, (11) _____ issues, and the limits of (12) _____.

Confidentiality is the principle that (13) _____ in therapy must be safeguarded by the therapist as (14) _____. With only a few exceptions, the content of therapy is considered (15) _____ communication, that is, the clinician may not disclose any information about the client without the client's (16) _____. Exceptions to this include instances involving (17) _____ reporting and duty to (18) _____. Mental health professionals are mandated by law to report information involving the (19) _____ or _____ of a child or people who are unable to (20) _____. The duty to warn involves the clinician's responsibility to take action to inform a (21) _____ of a client's (22) _____ to that person.

In their relationships with clients, clinicians must avoid (23) _____ relationships, such as (24) _____ with clients, and are expected to maintain (25) _____ and (26) _____ in their dealings with clients. Sometimes clinicians are called upon for special roles that present unique ethical challenges, such as being an (27) _____, preparing (28) _____ and evaluating people with (29) _____.

Clinicians are sometimes involved in the process of (30) _____, an emergency procedure for the involuntary hospitalization of a person deemed to be likely to create (31) _____ for self or (32) _____ as a result of (33) _____. Hospitalized clients have the right to a (34) _____ environment and to (35) _____ and (36) _____. Clients also have the right to refuse (37) _____ unless a court intervenes. Clients also have the right to be placed in the (38) _____ to treatment in an institution.

The major forensic issues that pertain to the field of mental health involve the (39) _____ and the competency to (40) _____. A client may plead insanity if, due to the existence of a (41) _____, he or she should not be held (42) _____ for (43)

_____ actions. The determination of competency to stand trial pertains to the question of whether a defendant is (44) _____ and able to (45) _____ criminal proceedings.

Multiple Choice

1. Which of the following is a guarantee that a clinician is capable of providing treatment to a client?
    a. A doctoral degree in clinical psychology
    b. A degree in medicine
    c. A state license to practice.
    d. None of the above.

2. Dr. Ward does not feel that she has the resources necessary to effectively treat Cindy's condition, and so she give Cindy the name and phone number of another clinician. Dr. Ward provided Cindy with
    a. informed consent.
    b. a referral.
    c. the right to refuse treatment.
    d. a mandated report.

3. Informing the client about the potential risks and benefits of therapy, confidentiality and its limits, and the expected length of therapy is necessary so that the client can
    a. understand his or her duty to warn.
    b. choose the least restrictive alternative.
    c. provide informed consent.
    d. establish commitment to therapy.

4. Nathan has been brought to the emergency room. He is extremely disoriented and is out of touch with reality. He has just attempted to commit suicide, and Dr. Gallina believes he is still at risk. Unfortunately, Nathan does not seem capable of providing informed consent for treatment. Dr. Gallina should
    a. respect Nathan's right to refuse treatment.
    b. get a court order to forcibly provide treatment.
    c. wait until Nathan becomes lucid.
    d. get consent from Nathan's family.

5. Why is confidentiality in therapy important?
    a. It is necessary in order for clients to feel comfortable disclosing intimate details about themselves during therapy.
    b. It is important for the clients to feel confident about improvement in their condition.
    c. It is a courtesy that has been brought about by the traditions of secrecy in the confessional.
    d. Most clients are collecting medical benefits and fear that if their bosses find out that they will lose the money.

6. Dr. Blanchard is being pressured by the local police department for information on one of his client's who is suspected of murder. Dr. Blanch must be careful to remember the principle of
    a. mandated reporting.
    b. privileged communication.
    c. informed consent.
    d. duty to warn.

7. The clinician's responsibility to notify a potential victim of a client's harmful intent toward that individual is referred to as
    a. primary prevention.
    b. notification of intent.
    c. duty to warn.
    d. legal commitment.

8. When a clinician is called on to provide specialized information not commonly known by people outside the mental health profession during court cases, he/she is considered to be a(n)
    a. *guardian ad litem.*
    b. expert witness.
    c. *parens patriae.*
    d. impartial party.

9. A person appointed by the court to represent or make decisions for a person who is legally incapable of doing so in a civil legal proceeding is referred to as a
    a. legal witness.
    b. *parens patriae.*
    c. parental authority.
    d. *guardian ad litem.*

10. If someone has not committed a crime but is viewed as being a potential threat to self or others, he or she may be
    a. involuntarily committed to a psychiatric hospital.
    b. judged incompetent to stand trial.
    c. judged as not guilty by reason of insanity.
    d. judged as guilty but insane.

11. The legal principle that the state has the authority to protect those who are unable to protect themselves is referred to as
    a. commitment.
    b. *guardian ad litem.*
    c. *ad hominen.*
    d. *parens patriae.*

12. Wendy has been involuntarily committed to a psychiatric hospital. When she tries to use the ward pay phone, the staff members stand nearby and listen to her conversation. Occasionally they have actually interrupted her calls and have hung the phone up on her. Which of Wendy's rights is being violated?
    a. the right to stand trial
    b. the right to treatment
    c. the right to a humane environment
    d. the right to refuse treatment

13. Which of the following is among the rights that apply to psychiatric patients?
    a. the right to refuse treatment
    b. the right to the most restrictive environment
    c. the right to legal counsel
    d. the right to die

14. Carol has been hospitalized after her most recent bout with depression which nearly resulted in her suicide. Her doctor insists that she receive electroconvulsive therapy. Despite the fact that she does not want the treatment, her doctor performs it anyway. Which of Carol's rights are being violated?
    a. the right to the least restrictive environment
    b. the right to refuse treatment
    c. the right to a humane environment
    d. the right to treatment

15. The subjective analysis of what the client would decide if he or she were cognitively capable of making the decision is
    a. *parens patriae.*
    b. *in loco parentis.*
    c. substituted judgement.
    d. informed consent.

16. What is the name of the rapidly growing subfield of psychology that examines issues pertaining to the relationship between criminal behavior and psychological disturbance?
    a. psychopathology
    b. clinical psychology
    c. forensic psychology
    d. legal psychology

17. Which of the following legal "tests" of insanity is based on the idea that people should not be judged guilty if a mental disorder prevents them from knowing the difference between right and wrong?
    a. the M'Naghten Rule
    b. the irresistible impulse test
    c. the Durham Rule
    d. the ALI guidelines

18. A person is not guilty if the "unlawful act was the product of mental disease or defect." This is the key feature of
    a. the M'Naghten Rule.
    b. the Durham Rule.
    c. the irresistible impulse test.
    d. the ALI guidelines.

19. What alternative verdict have some states utilized to separate the questions of guilt and mental disorder?
    a. not competent to stand trial
    b. the irresistible impulse verdict
    c. the least restrictive environment verdict
    d. the guilty, but mentally ill verdict

20. Which of the following individuals was found guilty, but insane, and sent to prison?
    a. Jeffrey Dahmer
    b. John Hinkley
    c. David Berkowitz
    d. Lorena Bobbitt

Answers

MATCHING

1. b	5. d	9. g
2. c	6. l	10. i
3. a	7. h	11. k
4. e	8. f	12. j

SHORT ANSWERS

1.
- a. The Insanity Defense Reform Act of 1984 had tightened the criteria for a person's psychological disorder to be regarded as grounds for insanity, partly in response to the criticisms of the outcome of the John Hinckley case. Further, Dahmer was diagnosed as having a sexual disorder but not a psychotic disorder unlike Hinckley.
- b. Legislation and judicial rulings regarding the determination of "insanity" focus on whether a person has the capacity to judge the rightness or wrongness of an act, to control his or her impulses to act, and appreciate the wrongfulness of an act.
- c. Determination of competency to stand trial involves predicting whether the defendant will have the cognitive capacity, emotional strength, and freedom from symptoms to make it possible to participate in court proceedings.
- d. Clinicians must determine whether the risk presented by a client to the self or others outweighs the client's right to live independently outside an institution.
- e. Clients are protected by the confidentiality of the clinician-client relationship, except when the clinician is obligated to follow through on a "duty to warn" another person about whom the client has expressed harmful intent or in cases where the client might inflict self-harm.
- f. Clients are entitled to provision of psychotherapeutic services; privacy; appropriate clothing; opportunities to interact with other people, to receive and send mail, to use the telephone, and to have visitation privileges; comfortable surroundings; exercise; and an adequate diet.

2.
- a. To provide relevant, professionally sound results or opinions in matters where a child's health may have been and/or may be harmed in the future
- b. The child's interest and well-being are paramount.
- c. The particular psychological and developmental needs of the child and/or parent(s) that are relevant to child protection issues such as physical abuse, sexual abuse, neglect, and/or serious emotional harm.
- d. Psychologists should provide an opinion regarding the psychological functioning of an individual only after conducting an evaluation of the individual adequate to support their statements or conclusions.
- e. Recommendations, if offered, are based on whether the child's health and welfare have been and/or may be seriously harmed.

3.
- a. Informed consent—the client must participate in setting treatment goals, understands and agrees to the treatment plan, and is aware of the clinician's credentials.
- b. Clinical interview and standardized psychological and neuropsychological tests.
- c. Constructive feedback, support, education, and a therapeutic alliance.

4.
- a. Those who were homeless experienced more hallucinations, persecutory delusions, emotional problems, impulsive behavior, and problems with alcohol and drug use, and were more likely to be noncompliant with their medications.
- b. Forty percent or more schizophrenic outpatients refuse medication or fail to take it as prescribed which they have the legal right to do. Treatment can be mandated only if they are a danger to themselves or others.

c. We need to know why clients who are schizophrenic refuse medication despite the sometimes dire consequences. Is it because it does not eliminate their symptoms or causes unpleasant side effects, or do they not appreciate its importance?

FOCUSING ON RESEARCH

1. A history of previous violence
2. Many factors can contribute to violent behavior including violent history, violent family background, history of drug abuse, being male, frequently moving, being unemployed, low intelligence, growing up in a violent subculture, and the availability of weapons and victims. However, many men with all of these factors don't commit violence. Thus, psychologists are reluctant to predict that men with these risk factors may be violent in the future. Further, not all men who are violent have these identifiable factors in their background, thus leaving open the possibility of false negatives (incorrectly predicting that someone won't be violent, when, in fact, they are) and false positives (incorrectly predicting that someone will be violent, when, in fact, they are not).
3. The clinician should (1) know what risk factors to look for in an assessment of a client's potential harm to others, such as previous history of violence and the base rate of specific types of violent crimes; (2) attempt to gather information about past treatment and arrests; (3) apply a prediction model that takes into account both demographic characteristics of the client and features of the client's particular disorder; and (4) ensure that this information is communicated to others and is documented in the client's records. Then preventive action can be taken, such as institutionalizing the client, warning the victim, and increasing contact with the client in the community.

FROM THE CASE FILES OF DR. SARAH TOBIN: THINKING ABOUT MARK'S CASE

1. When Dr. Tobin saw Mark in the Emergency Room, Mark was immobilized, in a catatonic state. He was unshaven, unkempt, and unresponsive to questions, but he suddenly grabbed a pen and gouged at his wrist. He did not appear to comprehend anything Dr. Tobin was saying. His wife reported that Mark had not eaten in days and was not sleeping much. He had recently urinated and defecated in his clothing, unaware that he was doing so. He was clearly a danger to himself.
2. Because of Mark's catatonic state, Dr. Tobin could not administer any assessment instruments. She had to rely on what she observed and what his wife reported about his recent history. She gave him the diagnosis of Major Depressive Disorder, Recurrent, with Catatonic Features.
3. Mark had a biological and psychological predisposition to a mood disorder. His mother suffered from recurrent depression, and some of Mark's experiences, such as the death of his father when he was only 5, and his inability to manage intense stress as he got older, were psychological factors contributing to his depression. He had struggled with depression for years and had a major episode in college. This time, his anxiety about being a parent seemed to trigger the depressive episode.
4. During Mark's hospitalization, he received six ECT treatments. He improved dramatically. He was discharged on antidepressant medication and had individual therapy with Dr. Tobin for 8 months. The therapy sessions focused on helping Mark develop strategies to minimize a relapse. Mark did fine until his son was born. He then became sad and tearful. Dr. Tobin saw him twice weekly for the next few weeks and increased the dosage of his antidepressant. Weekly sessions with Dr. Tobin resumed for another year; after which he saw her once a month, and eventually, twice yearly. He continued to take a low dose of antidepressant medication. He has been fine for several years.

REVIEW AT A GLANCE

1. assess
2. conceptualize
3. treat
4. informed consent
5. goals
6. therapy
7. rights
8. responsibilities
9. risks
10. techniques
11. financial
12. confidentiality
13. disclosures
14. private
15. privileged
16. consent
17. mandated
18. warn
19. abuse; neglect
20. protect themselves
21. possible victim
22. intention to do harm
23. inappropriate
24. sexual intimacy
25. neutrality
26. distance
27. expert witness

28. child custody
29. dementia
30. commitment
31. harm
32. other people
33. mental illness

34. humane
35. liberty
36. safety
37. unwanted treatment
38. least restrictive alternative
39. insanity defense

40. stand trial
41. mental disorder
42. legally responsible
43. criminal
44. aware of
45. participate in

MULTIPLE CHOICE

1. (d) is correct. Education (a and b) and licensing (c) are no guarantee of professional competence.

2. (b) is correct. (a) has to do with client consent to treatment; (c) the right of a hospitalized patient to refuse treatment; and (d) the requirements of mental health professionals to report certain types of abuse.

3. (c) is correct. (a) involves duty of a mental health professional to warn persons a client has threatened to harm; (b) involves the duty to provide the least intrusive treatment option; and (d) is determining if the client is committed to participating in treatment.

4. (d) is correct. (a) and (c) are incorrect because the professional must act if the client is a danger to himself; (b) is not necessary unless the family does not give consent.

5. (a) is correct. (c) is technically correct, but it is not why confidentiality is important; (b) and (d) have nothing to do with therapist-client confidentiality.

6. (b) is correct. Client confidentiality becomes a legal privilege if the client is involved in any legal proceeding; (a) involves duty to report certain types of abuse; (c) concerns the client's understanding of and agreement with treatment; and (d) involves a therapist's duty to warn people the client may have threatened to harm.

7. (c) is correct. (a) has nothing to do with responsibility to victims; (b) is not a term used in the context of treatment; and (d) are legal proceedings to protect a client who is a danger to himself or others.

8. (b) is correct. (a) involves being court-appointed to represent the interests of someone who cannot protect their legal interests; (c) is the doctrine that allows the government to intervene in a person's life in order to protect their well-being; and (d) has nothing to do with the described activity.

9. (d) is correct. (a) is irrelevant to the details; (b) is the doctrine that allows the government to intervene in a persons' life in order to protect their well-being; and (c) is not relevant to the described activity.

10. (a) is correct. (b), (c), and (d) would only become issues if someone had been charged with a crime.

11. (d) is correct. (a) involves the legal proceeding to get treatment for a person who is a danger to self or others; (b) is a person who protects the legal interests of persons who cannot do so for themselves; and (c) is a Latin term that has nothing to do with mental health treatment.

12. (c) is correct. (a), (b), and (d) are unrelated to the described scenario.

13. (a) is correct. (b) is the opposite of what patients are supposed to have; patients do not have (c) and (d).

14. (b) is correct. Carol has (a), (c), and (d), but they are not being violated in this scenario.

15. (c) is correct. (a) and (b) involve the government's rights to protect those who can't protect themselves; and (d) has to do with a client's knowledge of and consent to treatment.

16. (c) is correct. (d) is not a subfield; (a) is a term for mental illness; and (b) involves the treatment of mental illness.

17. (a) is correct. (b), (c), and (d) are variations the insanity defense.

18. (b) is correct. (a), (c), and (d) are variations of the insanity defense.

19. (d) is correct. (a) is not concerned with guilty or innocence; (b) is a variation of the insanity defense; and there is no such thing as (c).

20. (a) is correct. (b) and (d) were found not guilty by reason of insanity; and (c) was found guilty in spite of an insanity plea.